Depression and Heart Disease

T0340690

World Psychiatric Association titles in the "Depression" series

In recent years, there has been a growing awareness of the multiple interrelationships between depression and various physical diseases. This series of volumes dealing with the comorbidity of depression with diabetes, heart disease and cancer provides an update of currently available evidence on these interrelationships.

Depression and Diabetes

Edited by Wayne Katon, Mario Maj and Norman Sartorius
ISBN: 9780470688380

Depression and Heart Disease

Edited by Alexander Glassman, Mario Maj and Norman Sartorius
ISBN: 9780470710579

Depression and Cancer

Edited by David W. Kissane, Mario Maj and Norman Sartorius
ISBN: 9780470689660

Related WPA title on depression:

Depressive Disorders, 3e

Edited by Helen Herrman, Mario Maj and Norman Sartorius
ISBN: 9780470987209

For all other WPA titles published by John Wiley & Sons Ltd, please visit the following website pages:

http://eu.wiley.com/WileyCDA/Section/id-305609.html

http://eu.wiley.com/WileyCDA/Section/id-303180.html

Depression and Heart Disease

Editors

Alexander Glassman
*Department of Clinical Psychopharmacology,
New York State Psychiatric Institute, New York, NY, USA
and Department of Psychiatry, Columbia University
College of Physicians and Surgeons, New York, NY, USA*

Mario Maj
*Department of Psychiatry, University of Naples SUN,
Naples, Italy*

Norman Sartorius
*Association for the Improvement of Mental Health
Programmes, Geneva, Switzerland*

WILEY-BLACKWELL
A John Wiley & Sons, Ltd., Publication

This edition first published 2011 © 2011 John Wiley & Sons, Ltd.

Wiley-Blackwell is an imprint of John Wiley & Sons, formed by the merger of Wiley's global Scientific, Technical and Medical business with Blackwell Publishing.

Registered office: John Wiley & Sons Ltd, The Atrium, Southern Gate, Chichester, West Sussex, PO19 8SQ, UK

Other Editorial Offices:
9600 Garsington Road, Oxford, OX4 2DQ, UK
111 River Street, Hoboken, NJ 07030-5774, USA

For details of our global editorial offices, for customer services and for information about how to apply for permission to reuse the copyright material in this book please see our website at www.wiley.com/wiley-blackwell

The right of the author to be identified as the author of this work has been asserted in accordance with the UK Copyright, Designs and Patents Act 1988.

Library of Congress Cataloguing-in-Publication Data

Depression and heart disease / editors, Alexander Glassman, Mario Maj, Norman Sartorius.
    p. ; cm.
  Includes bibliographical references and index.
  ISBN 978-0-470-71057-9 (pbk.)
1. Depression, Mental–Complications. 2. Heart–Diseases–Psychological aspects. I. Glassman, Alexander H., 1934- II. Maj, Mario, 1953- III. Sartorius, N.
[DNLM: 1. Depressive Disorder–complications. 2. Depressive Disorder–psychology. 3. Cardiovascular Diseases–etiology. 4. Cardiovascular Diseases–psychology. WM 171]
RC537.D42746 2011
616.85'27–dc22

                                                                        2010027876

A catalogue record for this book is available from the British Library.

This book is published in the following electronic formats: ePDF ISBN 978-0-470-97229-8 Wiley Online Library ISBN 978-0-470-97230-4.

Set in 10/12 Pt Times by Thomson Digital, Noida, India.
Printed and bound in Singapore by Fabulous Printers Pte Ltd

First Impression 2011

Contents

List of Contributors

J. Thomas Bigger, Jr.   Department of Medicine, Columbia
University College of Physicians and Surgeons, New York, NY, USA

Robert M. Carney   Department of Psychiatry, Washington
University School of Medicine, St. Louis, MO, USA

Eco de Geus   Department of Biological Psychology,
VU University, Amsterdam, The Netherlands

Mary Kate Elfrey   Department of Medicine, Johns Hopkins
Bayview Medical Center, Baltimore, MD, USA

Kenneth E. Freedland   Department of Psychiatry, Washington
University School of Medicine, St. Louis, MO, USA

Alexander H. Glassman   Department of Clinical
Psychopharmacology, New York State Psychiatric Institute,
New York, NY, USA and Department of Psychiatry, Columbia
University College of Physicians and Surgeons, New York, NY, USA

Wei Jiang   Department of Psychiatry and Behavioral Sciences,
Department of Medicine, Duke South Hospital, Durham, NC, USA

Palmiero Monteleone   Department of Psychiatry, University of
Naples SUN, Naples, Italy

Glen L. Xiong   Department of Psychiatry and Behavioral Sciences,
Department of Medicine, University of California, Davis, CA, USA

Roy C. Ziegelstein   Department of Medicine, Johns Hopkins
Bayview Medical Center, Baltimore, MD, USA

Preface

The idea that depression is related to cardiac morbidity and death has been prevalent for hundreds of years. Although intuitively appealing, it has been scientifically difficult to prove. Both the existence of the association and the mechanisms behind the association have proven much more complicated than might have been expected. This book examines the evidence that the association exists, the various mechanisms that might underlie the association and our ability to treat depression in the face of cardiovascular disease.

Drs Jiang and Xiong review in their chapter the epidemiology of the comorbidity between depression and heart disease. Extensive epidemiological data is now available, but the interpretation of the data is complicated by the need to control for cardiac risk factors and medications that might be used to treat depression. Cigarette smoking is an example of a cardiac risk factor that is also known to be seen more frequently in depressed patients. From the perspective of depressed patients, it matters little if their risk for cardiac disease comes from cigarette smoking or is directly related to depression. However, this is an important distinction in any scientific understanding of the mechanisms creating the association.

Individuals suffering from depression followed for long periods of time are at excess risk for cardiac morbidity and mortality after controlling for treatment as well as known cardiovascular risk factors. Initially, studies focused on large community samples. This was done in order to avoid confounding with antidepressant medications, which were ubiquitous to samples collected from clinical populations, and because it minimised the possibility that depression was caused by chronic cardiac disease.

Since the 1990s, there has been a shift in interest from long-term studies of medically healthy individuals to the effects of depression in patients with known cardiovascular disease. Much of the interest has centred on the relationship between depression and acute coronary syndromes. The landmark study of Frasure-Smith in 1993 [1] indicated that depression observed in the cardiac intensive care unit predicted a fivefold increase in the risk of cardiac mortality over the next 6 months. Since that time a large number, but not all, studies have replicated this effect of depression. Many studies have controlled for both cardiac risk factors and the severity of the cardiac event and, although the effect size attributable to depression has diminished, the risk in depressed, post-coronary patients seems to exceed the increase in risk usually seen in physically healthy depressed individuals.

The high prevalence of depression, along with a higher risk associated with acute cardiac events, initially made it seem as if it would be relatively easy to study the influence of depression on both cardiac morbidity and mortality. However, a number of factors have conspired to make that task much more difficult than it originally seemed. Medical treatment of patients after an acute coronary syndrome has radically reduced the incidence of adverse cardiac events and, as a consequence of this, the number of depressed patients necessary to see an effect of antidepressant treatment on medical morbidity and mortality has increased. In addition, when studies began in the mid-1990s, the majority of cases of depression after an acute coronary syndrome were untreated. As the awareness of the risk associated with depression increased and information about the safety of selective serotonin reuptake inhibitors (SSRIs) grew, it became harder to find either ethics boards or depressed patients willing to accept placebo treatment. Although the need for a definitive clinical trial testing whether antidepressant treatment would reduce medical complications has been obvious for at least a decade, the cost and practicality of such a trial has grown more and more difficult.

While efforts to mount a definitive clinical trial have stalled, investigators have focused on potential mechanisms that might underlie the association between depression and heart disease. Health behaviours, compliance, platelet reactivity, heart rate variability, endothelial reactivity, sympathetic activity, genetics and inflammation have all been suggested as possible mediators. At this point it would seem very unlikely that any one mediator is responsible for the association. It is likely that the association stems from multiple sources and they are probably not the same in all depressed patients.

Drs Ziegelstein and Elfrey review in their chapter the behavioural and psychological mechanisms linking depression and heart disease, with a special focus on compliance with treatment. Statins, beta-blockers, anti-platelet drugs and calcium channel blockers reduce mortality after an acute coronary syndrome, but only if patients take their medication, and the evidence is that depressed patients are less likely to adhere to medical prescriptions. If treating depression successfully improves compliance, it must to some degree reduce morbidity and mortality. Although improved compliance and other health behaviours are almost certain to contribute to reducing the increased morbidity and mortality associated with depression, they will almost certainly account for only a part of the risk.

As reviewed by Dr Monteleone in his chapter, autonomic nervous system dysregulation, endothelial dysfunctions, platelet abnormalities, neuroendocrine abnormalities, and inflammation have all been suggested as potential biological mechanisms behind the association between depression and heart disease. All have been demonstrated to exist in both conditions. However, to which degree any of these potential mechanisms actually drive the association is unclear. Perhaps the best studied of these mechanisms involves inflammatory markers. Dozens of studies have looked for abnormal inflammatory markers in depressed patients and some markers are almost always found. The observation that alpha-interferon used to treat hepatitis C or malignant melanoma is associated with a marked increase in the onset of major depression makes it clear that increased inflammatory activity can provoke depression. However, it remains unclear whether inflammation associated with depression increases the risk of heart disease or if the degree of inflammation associated with acute heart disease increases the risk for depression. It is certainly possible that the relationship is bidirectional and/or that the inflammation characteristic of each condition is the result of some common genetic vulnerability. In a similar way, low heart rate variability is associated with increased mortality in cardiovascular patients and is also characteristic of more severe depressions and may be the result of some common genetic predisposition. The possible role of genetic factors in contributing to the association between depression and heart disease is reviewed by Dr de Geus in his chapter.

Regardless of the mechanism, a strong association between depression and the risk of cardiovascular morbidity and mortality makes the treatment of depression after an acute coronary syndrome all the more important. This became obvious in 1993 with the publication of Frasure-Smith's landmark paper. However, at that time, there was no evidence that antidepressant drugs were safe in the period immediately after an acute coronary syndrome. There was, in fact, considerable evidence that tricyclic antidepressants were dangerous in patients with cardiac disease. For that reason, the only large treatment trial of depression after an acute coronary syndrome compared psychotherapy with usual care. In that trial, psychotherapy was modestly more effective than usual care in reducing depression, but there was no evidence for any reduction in mortality. There is now a need to establish whether a more practical and efficacious psychotherapy can be developed. The other large trial was never powered to test the effect of antidepressants on medical risk, but was an SSRI safety trial. It was the early 2000s before it became clear that SSRIs were safe in the immediate period after an acute coronary syndrome. Interestingly, although the antidepressant effect was similar across drug and psychotherapy treatments, those patients who received an SSRI appeared to have a reduction in medical morbidity and mortality. Unfortunately, the evidence that SSRIs can reduce morbidity and mortality is suggestive but not definitive. Antidepressant use in the psychotherapy trial was not randomised and the SSRI treatment trial, although suggestive, was grossly underpowered to address the question. Current available evidence concerning pharmacotherapies and psychotherapies for depression in patients with heart disease is reviewed, respectively, by Drs Glassman and Bigger, and by Drs Carney and Freedland in their chapters.

Depression's importance as a public health problem is due to both its high lifetime prevalence and the significant disability that it causes. World Health Statistics in 2007 [2] revealed that individuals with depression and one other chronic condition had much lower health scores when compared with those who had only a chronic condition. Given that ischaemic heart disease and unipolar major depression are predicted by the World Health Organization to be the leading causes of disability-adjusted life years by 2020 [3], the increased risk associated with this comorbidity causes a dramatic increase in health burden worldwide. In many primary care settings, when patients present with multiple disorders that include depression, this condition often remains undiagnosed. Particularly in acute coronary events, even if it is diagnosed, treatment usually focuses on the coronary disease. The timely diagnosis and treatment of depressive disorders is essential, and understanding the mechanisms underlying the increased morbidity and mortality associated with the comorbidity of depression and heart disease is crucial to a rational treatment.

REFERENCES

1. Frasure-Smith, N., Lesperance, F. and Talajic, M. (1993) Depression following myocardial infarction. Impact on 6-month survival. *JAMA*, **270**, 1819–1825.
2. World Health Organization (2007) *World Health Statistics 2007*. World Health Organization, Geneva.
3. Mathers, C.D. and Loncar, D. (2006) Projection of global mortality and burden of disease from 2002 to 2030. *PLoS Med.*, **3**, 2011–2030.

Alexander Glassman
Mario Maj
Norman Sartorius

CHAPTER 1

Epidemiology of the Comorbidity between Depression and Heart Disease

Wei Jiang

Department of Psychiatry and Behavioral Sciences, Department of Medicine, Duke South Hospital, Durham, NC, USA

Glen L. Xiong

Department of Psychiatry and Behavioral Sciences, Department of Medicine, University of California, Davis, CA, USA

The relationship between mood states and the heart has been known since antiquity. Across various cultures, statements in present-day languages such as 'my heart aches' are used to communicate depressive emotions. Over the past three decades, a large body of evidence has emerged that documents the adverse impact of depressive disorders on cardiovascular disease. This confirms the early suspicion of astute clinicians that psychological factors play a significant role in the genesis and the course of heart disease, as well as the ancient belief in a mind–body connection in general and human moods and the heart in particular.

This chapter examines epidemiological studies that have investigated the relationship between depression and heart disease, with specific focus on the prevalence of depression in different populations

Depression and Heart Disease   Edited by Alexander Glassman, Mario Maj and Norman Sartorius
© 2011 John Wiley & Sons, Ltd

with cardiovascular disease and the adverse effects of depression on clinical outcomes.

We reviewed the literature through MEDLINE searches on English-language articles published between 1966 and September 2009 with the terms 'heart disease', 'ischaemic heart disease', 'myocardial infarction', 'coronary heart disease', 'heart failure', 'depression', 'depressive disorder' and 'antidepressants'. Because the heart diseases being investigated are almost exclusively cardiovascular, we use the term coronary artery disease (CAD) as a general descriptor unless otherwise specified. Depression is used as a general term for all depressive disorders and symptoms of depression.

DEPRESSION AFTER MYOCARDIAL INFARCTION OR UNSTABLE ANGINA

The incidence of major depressive disorder, as defined by DSM-III criteria, after myocardial infarction (MI) has been reported to be 16% by both Frasure-Smith et al. [1] and Schleifer et al. [2]. Other studies using similar diagnostic approaches have found rates up to 20% [3]. The rate of depression based on self-administered questionnaires has been generally higher and has varied among studies. In a study by Denollet and Brutsaert [4], the reported incidence of depression after MI was as high as 50.5%.

As noted in Table 1.1, the follow-up period to examine the relationship of depression and prognosis after MI commonly lasted 6–12 months. The mortality rates among clinically depressed patients were always significantly higher than those of clinically non-depressed patients. The relative risk ratio for death within 6 months among post-MI patients with versus without major depressive disorder was reported to be 3.1 by both Schleifer et al. [2] and Frasure-Smith et al. [1]. The results of 1-year follow-up varied (relative risk ratios from 2.3 to 7.5 across studies), possibly reflecting the different methods used to evaluate depression.

Frasure-Smith et al. [1] demonstrated that patients diagnosed with depression post MI were more than five times more likely to die from cardiac causes by 6 months than those without major depression. At 18 months, cardiac mortality had reached 20% in patients with major

Table 1.1 Depression and mortality of patients with recent myocardial infarction

	N	Female (%)	Depressed (%)/measures	Follow-up (mo)	RR*
Stern et al. [66]	68	19	22/Zung	12	7.5 (OR)
Schleifer et al. [2]	282	22	16/MDD (DSM-III)	6	3.1
Ahern et al. [67]	265	18	[+]/BDI	12	NA (p <0.05)
Ladwig et al. [68]	552	0	Severe/SIPI	6	4.9
			Moderate/SIPI		2.8
Frasure-Smith et al. [1]	222	22	16/MDD (DSM-IV)	6	3.1
Frasure-Smith et al. [5]	218	22	31.2/BDI score ≥10	18	6.64
Denollet and Brutsaert [4]	87	7	50.5/MBHI	7.9 yr	4.3
Frasure-Smith et al. [69]	896	31.6	32.4/BDI score ≥10	12	3.66
Kaufmann et al. [52]	361	31.6	27.2/DIS score ≥5	12	2.33
Irvine et al. [14]	671	17.2	Not reported/BDI score ≥10	24	2.45[a]
Lane et al. [12]	288	25	30.7/BDI score ≥10	12	**
Lauzon et al. [50]	587	21.1	35/BDI score ≥10	12	1.3
Grace et al. [16]	750	35	31.3/BDI score ≥10	60	1.90 (2 yr)
					2.53 (5 yr)
Parakh et al. [18]	284	43	26.8/BDI score ≥10	8 yr	0.6 (0.47, 1.24)
Carney et al. [70]	766	39.6	46.7[b]/BDI score ≥10	60	1.87 (1.17, 2.98)

* Adjusted relative risk ratio for mortality after myocardial infarction with versus without depression.
[+] Tested score differences between the dead and the survivors.
** Depressed not worse than non-depressed for mortality; depression predicted poorer quality of life.
[a] The increased RR only existed in placebo arm.
[b] Includes minor depression and dysthymia.
BDI – Beck Depression Inventory; MBHI – Millon Behavioural Health Inventory; MDD – major depressive disorder; SIPI – Standard Instruments of Psychological Inventory; DIS – Diagnostic Interview Schedule.

depression, compared with only 3% in non-depressed patients [5]. Recent work has confirmed and extended these findings. A meta-analysis of 22 studies of post-MI subjects found that post-MI depression was associated with a 2.0–2.5 increased risk of negative cardiovascular outcomes [6]. Another meta-analysis examining 20 studies of subjects with MI, coronary artery bypass graft (CABG), angioplasty or angiographically documented CAD found a twofold increased risk of death among depressed compared with non-depressed patients [7]. Though studies included in these meta-analyses had substantial methodological variability, the overall results were quite similar [8].

The impact of subclinical or minor depression (notable depressive symptoms, defined as a Beck Depression Inventory (BDI) score ≥ 10 but not meeting diagnostic criteria for major depressive disorder) on mortality after MI is no less than that of major depression [1, 2]. Frasure-Smith's group demonstrated that post-MI patients with a BDI score ≥ 10 were almost seven times more likely to die in the 18 months after their acute MI than were patients whose BDI score was <10 [5]. Such impact was independent of cardiac function, previous MI and frequency of premature ventricular arrhythmia, which are known risk factors for mortality in this population.

The time course of depression may be relevant in its relationship to CAD and cardiac morbidity. Post-MI depression includes both depression that pre-dated MI (non-incident depression) and depression that developed after MI (incident depression). In the Depression after Myocardial Infarction study, 25.4% of patients experienced depression during the year following MI, with 55.4% being non-incident episodes of depression [9]. Interestingly, those with incident depression had a trend towards a lower ejection fraction, increased disability at 12 months and a statistically higher risk of revascularisation. Incident post-MI depression was associated with new cardiovascular events in follow-up with a hazard ratio (HR) of 1.65 (95% CI 1.02, 2.65), whereas non-incident depression was not (HR 1.12, 95% CI 0.61, 2.06).

In another sample of patients ($N = 489$) hospitalised with acute coronary syndrome (ACS), the odds of being readmitted or dying were seven times higher for those with incident (post-ACS) depression [10]. Nevertheless, both incident and non-incident depression were found to increase the risks of cardiac death in the Enhancing Recovery In Coronary Heart Disease (ENRICHD) cohort with 1328 patients over 29 months. This study demonstrated that incident depression had higher risks of cardiac mortality (HR 3.1; 95% CI 1.6, 6.1) than recurrent depression (HR 2.2; 95% CI 1.1, 4) [11].

Of interest, a study from the UK by Lane et al. [12] reported that depression, defined as a BDI score ≥10, was not associated by logistic regression with increased mortality during 12-month follow-up, although it was associated with a further decline in quality of life [13]. The reliability of a self-administered questionnaire to assess true depression in a British population is unknown. Another recent study from the UK [13], using the Hospital Anxiety and Depression scale to measure depressive symptoms after MI, had similar results, that is no association with mortality but a negative association with poor quality of life [14]. Since the treatment of depression is not generally examined in these prospective studies, the impact of depression treatment on CAD outcomes may have contributed to different results in the various cohorts, with notable differences by country of study.

Irvine et al. [14], on the other hand, found that depression, defined as a BDI score ≥10, was associated with increased sudden cardiac death only in the placebo arm (RR 2.45; 95% CI 1.14, 5.35) during a 2-year follow-up, and not in the patients who received amiodarone for arrhythmia after MI. The size of the patient sample on amiodarone might have precluded the ability to detect a difference in this subgroup of patients.

Few studies have reported the relationship of depression with reinfarction or other outcomes such as unstable angina, heart failure or repeat hospitalisations after MI. Ladwig et al. [15] found that patients with depression after MI had an almost threefold higher risk of chest pain than non-depressed patients during 6-month follow-up. Although chest pain does not always reflect myocardial ischaemia, and depression has been considered to be associated with non-cardiac chest pain, any recurrent chest pain after MI warrants further evaluation.

The long-term (> 1 year) impact of major depression on mortality after MI has not been as well studied as the short-term one. Two recent studies report odds ratios of mortality at 5 years of 2.53 and 1.87 [16, 17]. There were two longitudinal follow-up studies examining the relationship of depression and survival after MI for 7.9 and 8 years, respectively. Denollet and Brutsaert [4] followed 87 Belgian patients for a mean 7.9 years (range 6–10 years) after MI. Depression was measured by the Millon Behavioural Health Inventory. How this inventory compares with those more frequently used in the literature is unknown. The relative risk ratio for cardiac death in the depressed patients was 4.3. The primary purpose of this study was to investigate the association of type D personality (tendency to suppress negative emotions) with mortality after MI; they did not report the independent ability of depression to predict survival. Parakh et al. [18] studied 284 patients using the BDI and found a prevalence of depression of 43% at Johns Hopkins Bayview Medical Center in Baltimore. They found that depression at the time of MI was not associated with mortality at 8 years (HR 0.76; 95% CI 0.47, 1.24). They concluded that the effect of depression after MI in increasing mortality seems to wane over time. However, this negative result might be due to the relatively small sample size. The most recent study involved 369 patients from the Sertraline AntiDepressant Heart Attack Trial (SADHART) cohort after 7 years of follow-up. Glassman et al. [19], using Cox proportional hazards regression models, found that baseline depression severity and failure of depression to improve substantially during treatment with either sertraline or placebo were strongly and independently associated with long-term mortality (HR 2.30; 95% CI 1.28, 4.14, and HR 2.39; 95% CI 1.39, 2.44, respectively).

DEPRESSION AND STABLE CORONARY ARTERY DISEASE

Of the patients with known CAD but no recent MI, 12–23% have major depressive disorder by DSM-III or DSM-IV criteria [20, 21]. Two studies have examined the prognostic association of depression in patients whose CAD was confirmed by angiography. Carney et al. [22] pioneered the studies in this area. In their study, a diagnosis of major depression by DSM-III criteria was the best predictor of cardiac events (MI, bypass surgery or death) at 1 year, more potent than other clinical risk factors such as impaired left ventricular function, severity of coronary disease and smoking among the 52 patients. The relative risk of a cardiac event was 2.2 times higher in patients with major depression than those with no depression. Mortality was not analysed separately from morbidity, most likely because of the small sample size.

Barefoot et al. [23] provided a larger sample size and longer follow-up duration in their study of 1250 patients who had undergone their first angiogram. They tested patients with the Zung Self-Rating Depression Scale (SDS) after angiography, then followed those with significant CAD ($\geq$75% diameter stenosis of at least one of the three major coronary arteries) for a mean of 19.4 years. A high SDS score was significantly associated with increased risks of cardiac death and all-cause mortality. Compared with non-depressed patients, those who were moderately to severely depressed had 69% higher odds of cardiac death and 78% higher odds of all-cause mortality. The mildly depressed had a 38% higher risk of cardiac death and a 57% higher risk of all-cause mortality than non-depressed patients. Of particular interest in this study is how the effect of depression on prognosis changed over time. During the first year of follow-up, the moderately to severely depressed patients had a 66% higher mortality rate than the non-depressed. This effect became somewhat weaker during years 2–5 of follow-up, but then re-emerged with an even greater association. The moderately to severely depressed patients had an 84% higher risk of mortality in years 6–10 than non-depressed patients, and a 72% higher risk beyond year 10 during the follow-up period. The persistent adverse impact of depression in CAD patients is consistent with the nature of depression, which is chronic, recurrent and fluctuating in severity. Unfortunately, the investigators did not report comorbidities such as reinfarction, revascularisations or repeat hospitalisations during follow-up.

More recently, studies have been extended to examine the prognostic impact of depression in other CAD populations. Lesperance et al. [24] studied 430 patients hospitalised for unstable angina without requirement for coronary artery bypass surgery. Among patients with a BDI score $\geq$10, the rate of death or MI 1 year after depression assessment was almost five times higher than their non-depressed counterparts. The association remained after controlling for other significant prognostic factors, including baseline electrocardiographic evidence of ischaemia, left ventricular ejection fraction and number of diseased coronary arteries (adjusted OR 6.73). The depressed patients were also more likely to be readmitted for unstable angina, although this finding did not reach statistical significance. There was no interaction between depression and percutaneous transluminal coronary angioplasty.

Although depression is less frequent among elderly people, the association of depression with adverse prognosis in CAD remains in old age. The Systolic Hypertension in the Elderly Program followed 4367 hypertensive subjects aged over 60 years for an average of 4.5 years and found an increased risk of death (RR 1.3), MI or stroke (RR 1.2) associated with the presence of significant depressive symptoms [25]. Furthermore, a study of 3701 subjects 70 years or older [26], followed for an average of 4 years, revealed that men with a new diagnosis of depression were about twice as likely to experience a cardiovascular event (RR 2.1) or die from cardiovascular causes (RR 1.8) than those without a history of depression.

DEPRESSION AND CORONARY ARTERY BYPASS GRAFTING

CABG surgery is frequently performed in patients with severe CAD. After a median follow-up of 9.4 years, surgical management compared favourably with medical treatment with respect to psychosocial outcomes, including lower depression and higher social functioning scores [27]. Nevertheless, adverse surgical outcomes following CABG in patients with depression were found in several studies [27, 28]. Patients with peri-operative depression or higher depressive symptoms experienced more recurrent angina and non-fatal cardiac events and higher mortality [29–31].

Although a large number of studies have examined the role of depression in post-MI and CAD outcomes, fewer studies have examined the role of incident and persistent depression on clinical outcomes after CABG (Table 1.2).

Early studies examined the role of emotional distress and depressive symptoms on CABG outcomes. Scheier et al. [29] used the Nottingham Health Profile and identified subjects who were in the 75th percentile in their severity of emotional distress before they underwent CABG. Over a follow-up period of 3 years, they found that

Table 1.2 Depression and clinical outcomes after coronary artery bypass grafting (CABG)

	N	Depression diagnosis and prevalence (%)	Timing of depression diagnosis	Follow-up	Outcome	Risk
Borowicz et al. [35]	172	CES-D ≥16 N = 55 (32%)	Before CABG, 1 mo, 1 yr, 5 yr	5 yr	Cardiac morbidity	CES-D ≥16 at 1 mo most predictive of chest pain
Peterson et al. [36]	N = 123	(New depression at 6 mo) CES-D ≥16 N = 12 (10%) Excluded initial CES-D ≥16 before CABG	6, 36 mo	36 mo	Composite (MI, shock, cardiopulmonary arrest, ARDS, pulmonary oedema, new angina, unstable angina)	OR 5.16 (0.97, 27.5)
Connerney et al. [34]	309	BDI N = 63 (20%)	After CABG, before discharge	12 mo	Angina or heart failure, MI, cardiac arrest, PCTA, redo CABG, cardiac death	HR 2.3 (1.17, 4.56)

(Continued)

Table 1.2 (Continued)

	N	Depression diagnosis and prevalence (%)	Timing of depression diagnosis	Follow-up	Outcome	Risk
Wellenium et al. [37]	1319	CES-D N = 127 (9.6%)	Enrolled 1–11 yr after CABG	4.2 yr	Graft disease progression	OR 1.50 (1.08, 2.10)
Burg et al. [28]	89	BDI N = 25 (28%)	Before CABG	24 mo 6 mo	Death Cardiac hospitalisation	OR 7.75**
Baker et al. [39]	158	DASS N = 25 (15.2%)	Before CABG	24 (3–38) months	Death	OR = 6.24 (1.18, 32.98)

| Blumenthal et al. [71] | 817 | CES-D N = 310 (38%) N = 97 (12%) moderate to severe (CES-D ≥27) | Before CABG, 6 mo Excluded patients with previous depression | Mean 5.2 yr Up to 12 yr | Death | Persistent depression HR 2.20 (1.17, 4.15) Moderate to severe depression 2.37 (1.40, 4) |

** Approximate calculations.
CES-D – Center for Epidemiologic Studies Depression Scale; BDI – Beck Depression Inventory; DASS – Depression Anxiety and Stress Scale; OR – odds ratio; HR – hazard ratio.

33 of 147 of those subjects had elevated rates of composite cardiac events, including CABG death, fatal MI, non-fatal MI, need for angioplasty and unstable angina [30]. Another early study examined optimism (10-item Revised Life Orientation Test) and found that it was associated with decreased hospital readmission after CABG [29]. Saur et al. [32] studied 416 subjects before CABG who reported the presence of depressive *symptoms* (using the Short-Form 36 Health Survey) and found that 'feeling down in the dumps' and overall mental health score correlated with hospital readmission within 6 months of CABG, but not with death. The studies cited above examined only depressive symptoms and did not explore whether depression was a disorder or episode (e.g. 2 weeks of continuous symptoms to be considered an episode as defined by the DSM-IV). In another more recent study, Tully et al. [33] found that anxiety symptoms seemed to be more predictive of mortality than depressive symptoms using the Depression Anxiety and Stress Scale in 440 pre-operative CABG patients. This study awaits further confirmation and is limited by the lack of a more rigorous diagnostic assessment.

Connerney et al. [34] published in 2001 the first study that specifically examined depression as a disorder using a structured psychiatric interview (Diagnostic Interview Schedule, DIS) and the BDI [34]. The subjects in the study were interviewed after CABG and followed up for 12 months. Of 309 participants, 63 (20%) met diagnostic criteria for major depression. The authors demonstrated that depression was associated with an HR of 2.3 (95% CI 1.17, 4.56) in composite outcomes of angina or heart failure, MI, cardiac arrest, need for angioplasty, need for redo CABG and cardiac death.

Soon after, Borowicz et al. [35] and Peterson et al. [36] monitored serial depression scores using the Center for Epidemiological Studies Depression Scale (CES-D). Borowicz et al. [35] examined 172 subjects and found that 32% of them were depressed pre-operatively, 28% were depressed at 1 month, 21% at 1 year and 16% at 5 years after CABG. The depression score at 1 month after CABG was an important indicator of cardiac morbidity up to 5 years. After multivariate analysis, an elevated CES-D score from the four time points (before CABG, 1 month, 1 year and 5 years) was most predictive of chest pain at 5 years, whereas other cardiac risk factors (male gender, smoking history, previous angioplasty and stroke) were not predictive. Peterson et al. [36] measured CES-D scores 6 and 36 months after CABG. After pre-operative screening, they excluded subjects who had CES-D scores ≥ 16 and recruited 123 subjects 6 months after CABG. The incidence of new depression at 6 months was 10%. Using a composite cardiac end point (new MI, shock, cardiopulmonary arrest, adult respiratory distress syndrome, pulmonary oedema, new-onset angina or unstable angina), the rate of events between 6 and 36 months was 13.6% among those with incident depression at 6 months versus 3.0% in the patients without new depressive symptoms at 6 months. Both of these studies were limited by their small samples sizes.

Wellenium et al. [37] conducted an intriguing study in 1319 patients 1–11 years after CABG and found that those who scored ≥ 16 on the CES-D had substantial risk of graft disease progression (OR 1.5; 95% CI 1.08, 2.10, $p = 0.02$). However, in patients who were assigned aggressive lipid-lowering therapy, the association was absent. This raises the interesting relationship between atherosclerosis and depression (since some have coined the term vascular depression) and the potential role of lipid reduction in depression modification [38].

Although the studies above did not examine mortality separately, a number of subsequent studies did. Burg et al. [28] examined 89 subjects with a depression prevalence of 28% before CABG and found that the OR for mortality post CABG at 2 years was 7.75. Baker et al. [39] studied 158 subjects with a depression prevalence of 15% before CABG and found a 2-year mortality odds ratio of 6.2. Thus, the findings from these studies, though conducted in different centres and countries, yielded similar risks of pre-operative depression for increased mortality after CABG. It is important to note that while the Burg study excluded subjects who also underwent concomitant valvular surgery, in the Baker study 134 underwent isolated CABG surgery and 24 underwent CABG surgery with a concomitant valve procedure.

Blumenthal et al. [31] published the largest cohort study (N = 817) to date on depression in patients undergoing CABG and measured depression scores, using the CES-D, before and at 6 months after CABG. Of those patients, 26% had minor depression (CES-D score 16–26) and 12% had moderate to severe depression (CES-D score ≥ 27). Over a mean follow-up of 5.2 years, the risk of death, compared with those without depression, was 2.4 (HR adjusted; 95% CI 1.4, 4.0) in patients with moderate to severe depression and 2.2 (95% CI 1.2, 4.2) in those whose depression persisted from baseline to follow-up at 6 months. This is one of the few studies that found a dose response (in terms of severity and duration) between depression and death in CABG in particular and in CAD in general.

DEPRESSION AND CORONARY ARTERY DISEASE DEVELOPMENT

Longitudinal cohort studies have empowered the search of whether depression plays a role in the aetiology of CAD. The preponderance of evidence strongly suggests that depression is a risk factor for CAD development. Table 1.3 summarises the results of large prospective or longitudinal studies that examined whether depression constitutes a risk factor for CAD [40, 41]. The common features of these studies include a large study population, at least part of which began without signs of CAD; relatively well-defined cardiac events; and statistically calculated odds ratios. Although there are concerns about the consistency of results for studies that have attempted to evaluate the ability of depression to predict CAD, the studies listed in Table 1.3 provide convincing evidence that depression does play an important aetiological role in CAD development.

The earliest longitudinal, large-sample study [42] indicated that depression may be associated with increased mortality from cardiovascular disease. The authors followed all patients (N = 8136) with a diagnosis of mood disorder admitted for the first time to Danish psychiatric hospitals from 1 April 1969 to 31 March 1976. During an average follow-up period of 4.25 years, they found the death rate from cardiovascular causes to be significantly higher (p <0.001) than the expected death rate.

In an observational study, Ford et al. [43] prospectively followed all male medical students who entered the Johns Hopkins Medical School from 1948 to 1964. At entry, the participants completed questionnaires about their personal and family history, health status and health behaviour, and underwent a standard medical examination. The cohort was then followed after graduation by mailed, annual questionnaires. The incidence of depression in this study was based on

Table 1.3 Depression and coronary artery disease development

Study	N	M/F	Measures	Follow-up (yr)	Events (n)	Type of events	Relative risk*
Hallstrom et al. [40]	1462	0/1462	Depression (psychiatric interview, DSM-III)	12	75	Nonfatal MI, angina, ischaemic ECG change	Severity of depression predicted angina only
Appels and Mulder [72]	3877	3877/0	Depression (Maastricht questionnaire)	4.5	59	MI (fatal = 21; non-fatal = 38)	2.28 for non-fatal MI; no association with fatal MI
Anda et al. [73]	2832	1345/1487	Depression affect, hopelessness (subscale of general well-being schedule)	12.4	189	Fatal MI	1.5, depression affect; 1.6, moderate hopelessness; 2.1, severe hopelessness
Aromaa et al. [74]	8000	2420/2935	Depression (GHQ, PSE)	6.6	91	Fatal CAD	3.36

(Continued)

Table 1.3 (Continued)

Study	N	M/F	Measures	Follow-up (yr)	Events (n)	Type of events	Relative risk*
Everson et al. [75]	2428	2428/0	Hopelessness	6	A. 87 B. 95	A. cardiovascular death B. MI	A. 2.52, moderate hopelessness; 3.9, high hopelessness B. 2.39, high hopelessness; increased but non-significant, moderate hopelessness
Wassertheil-Smoller et al. [25]		2053/2314	Depression (CES-D)	4.5	A. 355 B. 321 C. 126	A. All deaths B. MI or stroke C. MI	A. 1.26 B. 1.18 C. 1.14 but not significant
Barefoot and Schroll [76]	730	409/321	Depression (MMPI-obvious depression scale)	24	A. 290 B. 122	A. All deaths B. MI	A. 1.59 B. 1.71

Study	N	M/F	Depression measure	Follow-up (years)	N	Outcome	Risk estimate
Pratt et al. [77]	1551	583/968	Depression (psychiatric interview, DSM-III)	13	64	MI, self reported	4.54, major depressive episode 2.07, dysphoria
Ford et al. [43]	1190	1190/0	Depression (psychiatric diagnosis)	37	A. 103 B. 163	A. MI B. CAD	A and B: 2.12
Mendes de Leon et al. [48]	2812	945/1446	Depression (CES-D)	9	A. 255 B. 391	A. CAD death B. non-fatal MI, cardiac death	A and B: 1.03
Ariyo et al. [78]	4493	NA	Depression (CES-D)	6		A. CAD incidence B. All-mortality	A. 1.15 (every 5-point increase in CES-D scores) B. 1.29 (every 5-point increase in CES-D scores)
Ferketich et al. [79]	7893	2886/5007	Depression (CES-D)	10	A. 129/137 B. 187/187	A. CAD incidence M/F B. CAD death M/F	A. M 1.71/F 1.73 B. M 2.34/F 0.74 (95% CI 0.4, 1.48)

(Continued)

Table 1.3 (*Continued*)

Study	N	M/F	Measures	Follow-up (yr)	Events (n)	Type of events	Relative risk*
Penninx et al. [80]	2397	1091/13 065	Depression (DSM-III, CES-D)	4		Cardiac mortality	3.9, major depression 1.5 (95% CI 0.9–2.6), minor depression
Wassertheil-Smoller et al. [41]	93 676	0/93 676	CES-D	4.1	A. 18 572 B. 2306	A. CAD incidence B. MI	A. 1.41 (1.35–1.47) B. 1.45 (1.30–1.62) 1.58 (1.19–2.10) for cardiovascular death
Wulsin et al. [81]	3634	45%/55%	CES-D ≥ 16	6	A. 121 B. 133	A. CAD/cardiac death B. 133 all death	A. 0.64 (0.28–1.49) B. 1.50 (0.93–2.44)

Study	N	Method	Follow-up		Outcome	RR (95% CI)
Surtees et al. [82]	19 649 11 388/8261	DSM-IV criteria (structured self-assessment questionnaire)	8.5	274	Cardiac death	2.67 (1.54–4.64) both gender 2.05 (0.80–5.29) women 3.07 (1.55–6.08) men
Kendler et al. [83]	30 374 47.6%/53.4%	CIDI-SF	<1 yr and >1 yr		CAD incidence	2.53 (1.70–3.78) within 1 yr of major depression 1.17 (1.04–3.31) >1 yr of major depression

*Adjusted for multiple factors (various across studies, in general age, conventional cardiovascular risk factors such as smoking, cholesterol, weight or body mass index, and physical conditions at entry of the study).

CAD – coronary artery disease; CES-D – Center for Epidemiologic Studies Depression; GHQ – General Health Questionnaire; MI – myocardial infarction; MMPI – Minnesota Multiphasic Personality Inventory; PSE – Psychiatric State Examination; CIDS-SF – Composite International Diagnostic Interview-Short Form.

the mailed surveys, which asked direct questions about the occurrence of depression and associated treatment; a committee of five physician reviewers unaware of the study hypothesis confirmed the results. Depressive symptoms resolved within 2 weeks or symptoms related exclusively to grief were not considered 'depression' as a disorder for this study. Cardiovascular disease end points were collected by review of annual questionnaires, National Death Index searches, medical records, death certificates and autopsy records, which were then verified. The definition of CAD in this study included MI, angina pectoris, chronic heart disease and other types of symptomatic disease that did not meet these criteria but required CABG or percutaneous transluminal coronary angioplasty. Only very few participants were excluded for missing baseline information ($N = 59$) or for death during medical schooling or loss to follow-up ($N = 26$), leaving 1190 participants for analysis. The cumulative incidence of clinical depression in this population at 40 years of follow-up was 12%, with no evidence of a temporal change in the incidence. Less than a quarter of the clinically depressed participants received no treatment for depression; about a third used antidepressants and almost half received psychotherapy. In unadjusted analysis, clinical depression was associated with an almost twofold higher risk of subsequent CAD. This association remained after adjustment for time-dependent covariates such as smoking, alcohol use and coffee consumption. The relative risk ratio for CAD development with versus without clinical depression was 2.12 (95% CI 1.24, 3.63), as was their relative risk ratio for future MI (95% CI 1.11, 4.06), after adjustment for age, baseline serum cholesterol level, parental MI, physical activity, time-dependent smoking, hypertension and diabetes. The median time from the first episode of clinical depression to first CAD event was 15 years, with a range of 1–44 years. After excluding men whose CAD occurred within 2 years of clinical depression, to reduce the possibility that occult CAD might have existed before the onset of clinical depression, the repeated analysis revealed that the relative risk of CAD among depressed men remained significantly higher. This study has numerous strengths, including the prospective design, inclusive sample collection beginning at a relatively young age (average 26 years), long follow-up period with a high rate of compliance, objective verification of cardiovascular events and the use of clinical depression

rather than just depressive symptoms measured by self-rated questionnaires. However, this study was confined only to men, the majority
of them white (98%), who had a very narrow range of education, social
interaction and economic status. Furthermore, the diagnosis of clinical depression was based on self-report. Nevertheless, the lifetime rate
of depression (12%) in the study is almost identical to the rate (12.8%)
found in a sample of white men 45–55 years old who were represen-
tative of the US population [44].

Hallstrom et al. [40] gathered comprehensive medical and psychiatric examinations from a community sample of women in Gothenburg, Sweden, between 1968 and 1969. The psychiatric assessment
included a depression disorder assessment graded from 0 to 4, in
which a grade ≥ 2 corresponded to clinical depression, and the
Hamilton Rating Scale (HRS) score. These women were then followed for 12 years for the occurrence of angina pectoris, MI and death.
Higher values for both depressive disorder grade and HRS scores were
associated with a higher risk of angina pectoris. This all-female
sample provides compensatory data for that obtained by Ford
et al. [43] among men. The slight discrepancies between the studies
may reflect methodological differences in the Swedish study. This was
a rather young female population with respect to CAD prevalence: most
participants were 50 years old or younger, and only 11% were 54 years
old at enrolment. Major depressive disorder was diagnosed in only 55
of the total 795 women (7%). If most participants with major depressive
disorder had fallen into the younger groups, the chance of finding a
positive relationship between major depression and CAD would be
extremely reduced, given that the incidence of both angina pectoris and
MI were low (3.2% and 1.4%, respectively) in this population.

Although some studies have not found an association between
depression and CAD in women as they have in men, more recent
results indicate that such an association does exist for women [45]. In
the Women's Ischaemia Syndrome Evaluation (WISE) study, 505
women referred for coronary angiography were followed for a mean
of 4.9 years and completed the BDI [46]. Significantly increased
mortality and cardiovascular events were found among women
with elevated BDI scores, even after adjustment for age, cholesterol,
stenosis score on angiography, smoking, diabetes, education, hypertension and body mass index (RR 3.1; 95% CI 1.5, 6.3).

Some authors have contended that elevated depressive symptom scores may simply reflect generalised distress and not a true depressive disorder. The Stockholm Heart Epidemiology Program (SHEEP) study examined the risk of MI among subjects hospitalised for depressive disorder over a 26-year follow-up period [26]. This large population-based case-control study of 1799 cases and 2339 controls demonstrated a significantly increased risk for acute MI among subjects hospitalised for depression, even after controlling for confounding factors such as age, gender, smoking, physical activity and obesity. In fact, there might have been mildly depressed subjects who were not hospitalised and thus not identified as cases in this study, which would actually lead to an underestimation of the true effect of depression on future MI. Further compelling evidence comes from a meta-analysis of 28 studies comprising almost 80 000 subjects [47], which demonstrated that, despite heterogeneity and differences in study quality, depression was consistently associated with increased risk of cardiovascular diseases in general, including stroke. The strongest results were found for an increased risk of acute MI (RR 1.6) where there was less heterogeneity between studies.

Four studies have shown little or no association between depression and the development of CAD [25, 45, 48, 49]. These equivocal findings probably reflect variations in methods. Cross-sectional comparisons of samples are not as useful and reliable as longitudinal, prospective community studies to investigate the potential role of depression in the development of CAD. Furthermore, age, especially age at entry in relation to sex, has been shown to substantially affect this assessment.

In Canada, Lauzon et al. [50] followed 587 patients from five tertiary and five community hospitals and examined depression using the BDI. They found that depressed patients were more likely to undergo cardiac catheterisation (57% vs 47%), and were more likely to undergo percutaneous coronary intervention (32% vs 24%) within 30 days of first admission to hospital. Patients with depression on admission had higher rates of a composite of cardiac complications, including recurrent ischaemia, infarction or congestive heart failure during their first stay in hospital or readmission for angina, recurrent acute MI, congestive heart failure or arrhythmia, than patients who were not depressed on admission. Other similar studies have also found increased health services use in depressed patients after ACS compared with non-depressed control subjects [51].

In summary, it is fair to conclude that depression plays a significant role in CAD development, independent of conventional risk factors, and its adverse impact endures over time. The impact of depression on the risk of MI is probably similar to that of smoking [52]. A commonly raised philosophical question is 'which came first, the chicken or the egg?'. Results of longitudinal cohort studies suggest that depression occurs before the onset of clinically significant CAD, but atherosclerosis, the underlying pathological process of CAD, is known to begin at very young ages. The fibrous plaque, an advanced lesion of atherosclerosis, generally appears during early adulthood [53]. Recent brain imaging studies have indicated that lesions resulting from cerebrovascular insufficiency may lead to clinical depression [54, 55]. Depression may be a clinical manifestation of atherosclerotic lesions in certain areas of the brain that cause circulatory deficits. The depression then exacerbates the onset of CAD. The exact aetiological mechanism of depression and CAD development remains to be clarified.

DEPRESSION AND CONGESTIVE HEART FAILURE

Few studies have examined the relationship between depression and heart diseases other than CAD. Studies aiming at exploring the relation between depression and congestive heart failure (CHF) did not begin until the 1990s, which was probably related to the increased recognition of depression impact in CAD and the increased negative impact of CHF. This has become a major public health problem over two to three decades, partly because of extended life expectancies and significant reductions in mortality from ACS. According to the National Heart, Lung, and Blood Institute [56], more than 2 million Americans have CHF, and about 400 000 new cases are diagnosed each year. The disorder carries an average 1-year mortality rate of about 10%, increasing to 50% at 5 years after diagnosis. Further, the rehospitalisation rate is 25–50% within 3–6 months [57, 58].

In an early attempt to examine whether depression may further increase the already high mortality in CHF patients, three studies

Table 1.4 Depression and heart failure

Author	N	Prevalence of depression (%)	Depression measures	Follow-up (yr)	Type of events	Relative risk*
Freedland et al. [61]	60	17.0	DSM-III	1	Death, hospitalisation	1.71 (0.80–3.67)
Krumholz et al. [59]	292	Not stated	CES-D	1	Death, hospitalisation	Depression: not associated with death. Lack of emotional support: associated with increased risk of death (OR 3.2, 95% CI 1, 7.8)
Murberg et al. [63]	119	Not stated	ZDS	2	Death	Depressed mood predicted death: HR 1.9, p = 0.002

Jiang et al. [62]	374	BDI: 35.3, MDD: 13.9	BDI DSM-IV	1	Death, hospitalisation	Death: 3-month: OR 2.5, p = 0.08; 1-year: OR 2.23, p = 0.04; Hospitalisation: 3-month: OR 1.9, p = 0.04; 1-year: OR 3.07, p = 0.005
Vaccarino et al. [64]	391	Mild: 35 Moderate: 33.5 Severe: 9.0	GDS	0.5	Death	Death rate: Normal 11.4%; Mild 16.1%; Moderate 22.1%; Severe 25.7%
Faris et al. [84]	396	21	Medical record	5	Death, hospitalisation, cardiac transplant	Death: HR 3.0, p = 0.004 Hospitalisation: HR 0.25, p = 0.03
de Denus et al. [85]	171	20	Medical record	0.63	Combined end point of in-hospital, death or CPR	Combined end point: OR 3.3, p <0.05

(Continued)

Table 1.4 (Continued)

Author	N	Prevalence of depression (%)	Depression measures	Follow-up (yr)	Type of events	Relative risk*
Sullivan et al. [86]	142	29	DSM-IV	3	Combined end point of death or transplant	Combined: 2.54, p=0.019; Transplant: 3.29, p=0.01; Death: 1.65, p=0.4
Junger et al. [87]	209	Not stated	HADS ≥8	2	Death	RR 8.2; 95% CI 2.62, 25.84
Friedmann et al. [88]	153	36	BDI >13	2	Death	1.81, p <0.04
Jiang et al. [89]	1006	30	BDI >9	2.6	Death	HR 1.36; CI 1.09, 1.70
Sherwood et al. [90]	204	46.1	BDI	3	Death or cardiac hospitalisation	Combined: HR 1.56; 95% CI 1.07, 2.29
Macchia et al. [91]	48 117	6.9	Antidepressant use	1	Death, cardiac event	Death: HR 1.20, p <0.001; Composite cardiac event: HR 1.23, p <0.001

Parissis et al. [92]	155	49	BDI ZDS	Death or CHF hospitalisation	0.5	ZDS score predicted combined end point of death or hospitalisation: 'area under curve' (AUC) = 0.683, p <0.01; BDI did not predict: AUC = 0.605, p = 0.05
Albert et al. [93]	48 612	10.6	Medical records	Death	0.08	HR 1.10, p = 0.035
Schiffer et al. [94]	366	Not stated	BDI	Death	3	Somatic and depressive symptoms: HR 2.3, p = 0.001; depressive symptoms: HR 1.6, p <0.05

BDI – Beck Depression Inventory; CHF – Congestive Heart Failure; HR – hazard ratio; CES-D – Center for Epidemiological Studies Depression Scale; GDS – Geriatric Depression Scale; ZDS – Zung Depression Scale.

failed to show that depression was associated with an increased risk of mortality in patients with CHF [59–61]. In a study by Krumholz et al. [59], depression was assessed before the diagnosis of CHF. Although depression was not associated with poorer prognosis in that study, a lack of emotional support, which relates significantly to the occurrence of depression, was an independent risk factor for increased mortality at 1 year after CHF diagnosis. The critical drawback of this study is that 37% of patients were excluded from follow-up because they did not meet criteria for major, minor or no depression, thus losing the features of a cohort study.

We conducted a prospective cohort study to examine whether depression adversely affects prognosis in CHF similarly to its effects in CAD and, if so, whether such effects occur independent of traditional risk factors. We also questioned whether an ischaemic aetiology of CHF makes patients more prone to depression and whether depression interacts with severity of cardiac dysfunction. We tested for depression 374 patients hospitalised with New York Heart Association class $\geq$II CHF and followed them for 12 months. Contrary to findings of previous studies, patients who met DSM-IV criteria for major depression had a mortality rate more than twice that of those who were not depressed, and three times as many rehospitalisations. These associations were present at 3 months and persisted through 1 year. Although advanced age and ischaemic aetiology of CHF were associated with increased mortality, the adverse relation of depression to mortality and morbidity was independent of these factors. A higher rate of depression was observed in patients with poorer cardiac function, but depression was not more prevalent among CHF patients with an ischaemic versus non-ischaemic aetiology [62].

Around a similar time, Murberg et al. [63] published their study that followed 119 clinically stable CHF patients for 24 months after assessing their depressed mood with Zung scale. They found that depressed mood was a significant predictor of mortality with a HR of 1.9 (p $=$ 0.002). Vaccarino et al. [64] measured the level of depressive symptoms by means of the Geriatric Depression Scale (GDS) among a group of patients (N $=$ 391) aged 50 or older who were hospitalised with CHF. They followed the patients for 6 months and measured their functional capacity, as activities of daily living (ADL), and the rate of death. They found that mortality at 6 months was 2–3 times higher in patients with greater depressive symptoms compared with patients with lesser depressive symptoms or patients considered to have normal mood. Patients with moderate to severe depressive symptoms also had significant functional declines during the follow-up period. Covariate adjustment for age, sex, race, and education appeared not to affect the relationship of depression to mortality or functional decline, but additional adjustment for prior MI, diabetes, previous admission for CHF, certain limiting factors of ADL, and a group of clinical features on presentation (systolic blood pressure, serum creatinine, pulse and left ventricular ejection fraction) eliminated the adverse relation of depression to mortality. The adverse effects of moderate depression on functional decline also were diminished. These results bring up two concerns. First, GDS is a valid measure for depressive symptoms among the elderly but is not equivalent to a clinical diagnosis of depression through standard diagnostic interviewing. Second, the number of variables to include as adjustment factors, given the number of events, and what potential confounding factors must be examined through statistical analysis remain challenging questions.

A number of studies in similar populations have been published since supporting our findings (Table 1.4). Rutledge et al. [65] conducted a meta-analysis in 2006 in order to better understand the prevalence of depression among patients with CHF and the magnitude of the relationship between depression and clinical outcomes in the CHF population. They found that clinically significant depression was present in 21.5% of CHF patients, varying by the use of questionnaires versus diagnostic interview (33.6% and 19.3%, respectively). The combined results suggested higher rates of death and secondary events (RR 2.1; 95% CI 1.7, 2.6), and trends toward increased health care use and higher rates of hospitalisation and emergency room visits among depressed patients. The results of the meta-analysis consolidated the evidence demonstrating depression as a risk of CHF.

CONCLUSIONS AND CLINICAL IMPLICATIONS

Depression is relatively prevalent among patients with heart disease, and it has a significant adverse relationship with CAD development and the prognosis of CAD and CHF. With the inability to identify the onset of atherosclerosis in relation to the onset of depression, the issue of 'which came first, the chicken or the egg' remains open.

The overriding imperative should be to recognise depression as early as possible and intervene appropriately. The underlying patho-physiological mechanisms of depression and its impact on cardiovascular disease as well as appropriate management of depression are discussed in other chapters of the book. Of critical importance is investigation into whether treatment of depression can improve the poorer prognosis in patients with heart disease.

REFERENCES

1. Frasure-Smith, N., Lesperance, F. and Talajic, M. (1993) Depression following myocardial infarction. Impact on 6-month survival. *JAMA*, **270,** 1819–1825.

2. Schleifer, S.J., Macari-Hinson, M.M., Coyle, D.A. et al. (1989) The nature and course of depression following myocardial infarction. *Arch. Intern. Med.*, **149,** 1785–1789.

3. Thombs, B.D., Bass, E.B., Ford, D.E. et al. (2006) Prevalence of depression in survivors of acute myocardial infarction. *J. Gen. Intern. Med.*, **21,** 30–38.

4. Denollet, J. and Brutsaert, D.L. (1998) Personality, disease severity, and the risk of long-term cardiac events in patients with a decreased ejection fraction after myocardial infarction. *Circulation*, **97,** 167–173.

5. Frasure-Smith, N., Lesperance, F. and Talajic, M. (1995) Depression and 18-month prognosis after myocardial infarction. *Circulation*, **91,** 999–1005.

6. Van Melle, J.P., de Jonge, P., Spijkerman, T.A. et al. (2004) Prognostic association of depression following myocardial infarction with mortality and cardiovascular events: a meta-analysis. *Psychosom. Med.*, **66,** 814–822.

7. Barth, J., Shumacher, M. and Hermann-Lingen, C. (2004) Depression as a risk factor for mortality in patients with coronary heart disease: a meta-analysis. *Psychosom. Med.*, **66,** 802–813.

8. Bush, D.E., Ziegelstein, R.C., Patel, U.V. et al. (2005) Post-myocardial infarction depression. *Evid. Rep. Technol. Assess.*, **123,** 1–8.

9. De Jonge, P., van den Brink, R.H.S., Spijkerman, T.A. and Ormel, J. (2006) Only incident depressive episodes after myocardial infarction are associated with new cardiovascular events. *J. Am. Coll. Cardiol.*, **48,** 2204–2208.

10. Parker, G.B., Hilton, T.M., Walsh, W.F. et al. (2008) Timing is everything: the onset of depression and acute coronary syndrome outcome. *Biol. Psychiatry.*, **64,** 660–666.

11. Carney, R.M., Freeland, K.E., Steinmeyer, B. et al. (2009) History of depression and survival after acute myocardial infarction. *Psychosom. Med.*, **71,** 253–259.

12. Lane, D., Carroll, D., Ring, C. et al. (2001) Mortality and quality of life after myocardial infarction: effects of depression and anxiety. *Psychosom. Med.*, **63,** 221–230.

13. Mayou, R.A., Gill, D., Thompson, D.R. et al. (2000) Depression and anxiety as predictors of outcome after myocardial infarction. *Psychosom. Med.*, **62,** 212–219.

14. Irvine, J., Basinski, A., Baker, B. et al. (1999) Depression and risk of sudden cardiac death after acute myocardial infarction: testing for the confounding effects of fatigue. *Psychosom. Med.*, **61,** 729–737.

15. Ladwig, K.H., Roll, G., Breithardt, G. and Borggrefe, M. (1999) Extracardiac contributions to chest pain perception in patients 6 months after acute myocardial infarction. *Am. Heart J.*, **137,** 528–535.

16. Grace, S., Abbey, S., Kapral, M. et al. (2005) Effect of depression on five-year mortality after an acute coronary syndrome. *Am. J. Cardiol.*, **96,** 1179–1185.

17. Carney, R.M., Freedland, K.E., Steinmeyer, B. et al. (2009) History of depression and survival after acute myocardial infarction. *Psychosom. Med.*, **71,** 253–259.

18. Parakh, K., Thombs, B.D., Fauerbach, A.J. et al. (2008) Effect of depression on late (8 years) mortality after myocardial infarction. *Am. J. Cardiol.*, **101,** 602–606.

19. Glassman, A.H., Bigger, J.T. and Gaffney, M. (2009) Psychiatric characteristics associated with long-term mortality among 361 patients having an acute coronary syndrome and major depression: seven-year follow-up of SADHART participants. *Arch. Gen. Psychiatry*, **66,** 1022–1029.

20. Carney, R.M., Freedland, K.E., Eisen, S.A. et al. (1995) Major depression and medication adherence in elderly patients with coronary artery disease. *Health Psychol.*, **14,** 88–90.

21. Sullivan, M., LaCroix, A., Russo, J. et al. (1999) Depression in coronary heart disease. What is the appropriate diagnostic threshold? *Psychosomatics*, **40,** 286–292.

22. Carney, R.M., Rich, M.W., Freedland, K.E. et al. (1988) Major depressive disorder predicts cardiac events in patients with coronary artery disease. *Psychosom. Med.*, **50,** 627–633.

23. Barefoot, J.C., Helms, M.J., Mark, D.B. et al. (1996) Depression and long-term mortality risk in patients with coronary artery disease. *Am. J. Cardiol.*, **78,** 613–617.

24. Lesperance, F., Frasure-Smith, N., Juneau, M. and Theroux, P. (2000) Depression and 1-year prognosis in unstable angina. *Arch. Intern. Med.*, **160,** 1354–1360.

25. Wassertheil-Smoller, S., Applegate, W.B., Berge, K. et al. (1996) Change in depression as a precursor of cardiovascular events. *Arch. Intern. Med.*, **156,** 553–561.

26. Penninx, B.W., Guralnik, J.M., Mendes de Leon, C.F. et al. (1998) Cardiovascular events and mortality in newly and chronically depressed persons > 70 years of age. *Am. J. Cardiol.*, **81,** 988–994.

27. Ben-Noun, L. (1999) Coronary artery bypass grafting: long-term psychological and social outcomes. *J. Anxiety Disord.*, **13,** 505–512.

28. Burg, M.M., Benedetto, M.C., Rosenberg, R.A. and Soufer, R. (2003) Presurgical depression predicts medical morbidity 6 months after coronary artery bypass graft surgery. *Psychosom. Med.*, **65,** 111–118.

29. Scheier, M.F., Matthew, K.A., Owens, J.F. et al. (1999) Optimism and rehospitalization after coronary artery bypass graft surgery. *Arch. Intern. Med.*, **159,** 829–835.

30. Perski, A., Feleke, E., Anderson, G. et al. (1998) Emotional distress before coronary bypass grafting limits the benefits of surgery. *Am. Heart J.*, **136,** 510–517.

31. Blumenthal, J.A., Lett, H.S., Babyak, M.A. et al. (2003) Depression as a risk factor for mortality after coronary artery bypass surgery. *Lancet*, **362,** 604–609.

32. Saur, C.D., Granger, B.B., Muhlbaier, L.H. et al. (2001) Depressive symptoms and outcome of coronary artery bypass grafting. *Am. J. Crit. Care*, **10,** 4–10.

33. Tully, P.J., Baker, R.A. and Knight, J.L. (2008) Anxiety and depression as risk factors for mortality after coronary artery bypass surgery. *J. Psychosom. Res.*, **64,** 285–290.

34. Connerney, I., Shapiro, P.A., McLaughlin, J.S. et al. (2001) Relation between depression after coronary artery bypass surgery and 12-month outcome: a prospective study. *Lancet*, **358,** 1766–1771.

35. Borowicz, L. Jr., Royall, R., Grega, M. et al. (2002) Depression and cardiac morbidity 5 years after coronary artery bypass surgery. *Psychosomatics*, **43,** 464–471.

36. Peterson, J.C., Charlson, M.E., Williams-Russo, P. et al. (2002) New postoperative depressive symptoms and long-term cardiac outcomes

after coronary artery bypass surgery. *Am. J. Geriatr. Psychiatry*, **10**, 192–198.

37. Wellenium, G.A., Mukamal, K.J., Kulshreshtha, A. et al. (2008) Depressive symptoms and the risk of atherosclerotic progression among patients with coronary artery bypass grafts. *Circulation*, **117**, 2313–2319.

38. Alexopoulos, G.S. (2006) The vascular depression hypothesis: 10 years later. *Biol. Psychiatry*, **60**, 1306–1308.

39. Baker, R.A., Andrew, M.J., Schrader, G. and Knight, J.L. (2001) Preoperative depression and mortality in coronary artery bypass surgery: preliminary findings. *Aust. N.Z. J. Surg.*, **71**, 139–142.

40. Hallstrom, T., Lapidus, L., Bengtsson, C. and Edstrom, K. (1986) Psychosocial factors and risk of ischaemic heart disease and death in women: a twelve-year follow-up of participants in the population study of women in Gothenburg, Sweden. *J. Psychosom. Res.*, **30**, 451–459.

41. Wassertheil-Smoller, S., Shumaker, S., Ockene, J. et al. (2004) Depression and cardiovascular sequelae in postmenopausal women: the Women's Health Initiative. *Arch. Intern. Med.*, **164**, 289–298.

42. Weeke, A., Juel, K. and Vaeth, M. (1987) Cardiovascular death and manic-depressive psychosis. *J. Affect. Disord.*, **13**, 287–292.

43. Ford, D.E., Mead, L.A., Chang, P.P. et al. (1998) Depression is a risk factor for coronary artery disease in men: the Precursors study. *Arch. Intern. Med.*, **158**, 1422–1426.

44. Blazer, D.G., Kessler, R.C., McGonagle, K.A. and Swartz, M.S. (1994) The prevalence and distribution of major depression in a national community sample: the National Comorbidity Survey. *Am. J. Psychiatry*, **151**, 979–986.

45. Goldberg, E.L., Comstock, G.W. and Hornstra, R.K. (1979) Depressed mood and subsequent physical illness. *Am. J. Psychiatry*, **136**, 530–534.

46. Rutledge, T., Reis, S.E., Olson, M.B. et al. (2006) Depression symptom severity and reported treatment history in the prediction of cardiac risk in women with suspected myocardial ischemia. *Arch. Gen. Psychiatry*, **63**, 874–880.

47. Van der Kooy, K., van Hout, H., Marwijk, H. et al. (2007) Depression and the risk for cardiovascular diseases: systematic review and meta analysis. *Int. J. Geriatr. Psychiatry*, **22**, 613–626.

48. Mendes de Leon, C.F., Krumholz, H.M., Seeman, T.S. et al. (1998) Depression and risk of coronary heart disease in elderly men and women: New Haven EPESE, 1982–1991. Established Populations for the Epidemiologic Studies of the Elderly. *Arch. Intern. Med.*, **158**, 2341–2348.

49. Vogt, T., Pope, C., Mullooly, J. and Hollis, J. (1994) Mental health status as a predictor of morbidity and mortality: a 15-year follow-up of members of a health maintenance organization. *Am. J. Publ. Health*, **84,** 227–231.

50. Lauzon, C., Beck, C.A., Huynh, T. et al. (2003) Depression and prognosis following hospital admission because of acute myocardial infarction. *CMAJ*, **168,** 547–552.

51. Kurdyak, P.A., Gnam, W.H. and Goering, P. (2008) The relationship between depressive symptoms, health service consumption, and prognosis after acute myocardial infarction: a prospective cohort study. *BMC Health Serv. Res.*, **8,** 200.

52. Kaufman, D.W., Helmrich, S.P., Rosenberg, L. et al. (1983) Nicotine and carbon monoxide content of cigarette smoke and the risk of myocardial infarction in young men. *N. Engl. J. Med.*, **308,** 409–413.

53. Stary, H.C. (1989) Evolution and progression of atherosclerotic lesions in coronary arteries of children and young adults. *Arteriosclerosis*, **9,** I19–I22.

54. Krishnan, K.R., Hays, J.C. and Blazer, D.G. (1997) MRI-defined vascular depression. *Am. J. Psychiatry*, **154,** 497–501.

55. Doraiswamy, P.M., MacFall, J., Krishnan, K.R. et al. (1999) Magnetic resonance assessment of cerebral perfusion in depressed cardiac patients: preliminary findings. *Am. J. Psychiatry*, **156,** 1641–1643.

56. Konstam, M.A., Dracup, K., Baker, D. et al. (1994) *Heart failure: evaluation and care of patients with left-ventricular dysfunction.* Clinical Practice Guideline No. 11. 1–21.

57. Gooding, J. and Jette, A.M. (1985) Hospital readmissions among the elderly. *J. Am. Geriatr. Soc.*, **33,** 595–601.

58. Vinson, J.M., Rich, M.W., Sperry, J.C. et al. (1990) Early readmission of elderly patients with congestive heart failure. *J. Am. Geriatr. Soc.*, **38,** 1290–1295.

59. Krumholz, H.M., Butler, J., Miller, J. et al. (1998) Prognostic importance of emotional support for elderly patients hospitalized with heart failure. *Circulation*, **97,** 958–964.

60. Koenig, H.G. (1998) Depression in hospitalized older patients with congestive heart failure. *Gen. Hosp. Psychiatry*, **20,** 29–43.

61. Freedland, K., Carney, R., Rich, M. and Caracciolo, A. (1991) Depression in elderly patients with congestive heart failure. *J. Geri. Psychiatry*, **24,** 59–71.

62. Jiang, W., Alexander, J., Christopher, E. et al. (2001) Relationship of depression to increased risk of mortality and rehospitalization in patients with congestive heart failure. *Arch. Intern. Med.*, **161,** 1849–1856.

63. Murberg, T.A., Bru, E., Svebak, S. et al. (1999) Depressed mood and subjective health symptoms as predictors of mortality in patients with congestive heart failure: a two-years follow-up study. *Int. J. Psychiatry Med.*, **29,** 311–326.
64. Vaccarino, V., Kasl, S.V., Abramson, J. and Krumholz, H.M. (2001) Depression symptoms and risk of functional decline and death in patients with heart failure. *J. Am. Coll. Cardiol.*, **38,** 199–205.
65. Rutledge, T., Reis, V., Linke, S. et al. (2006) Depression in heart failure: a meta-analytics review of prevalence, intervention effects, and associations with clinical outcomes. *J. Am. Coll. Cardiol.*, **48,** 1527–1537.
66. Stern, M.J., Pascale, L. and Ackerman, A. (1977) Life adjustment postmyocardial infarction: determining predictive variables. *Arch. Intern. Med.*, **137,** 1680–1685.
67. Ahern, D.K., Gorkin, L., Anderson, J.L. et al. (1990) Biobehavioral variables and mortality or cardiac arrest in the Cardiac Arrhythmia Pilot Study (CAPS). *Am. J. Cardiol.*, **66,** 59–62.
68. Ladwig, K.H., Roll, G., Breithardt, G. et al. (1994) Post-infarction depression and incomplete recovery 6 months after acute myocardial infarction. *Lancet*, **343,** 20–23.
69. Frasure-Smith, N., Lesperance, F., Juneau, M. et al. (1999) Gender, depression, and one-year prognosis after myocardial infarction. *Psychosom. Med.*, **61,** 26–37.
70. Carney, R., Freedland, K., Steinmeyer, B. et al. (2008) Depression and five year survival following acute myocardial infarction: a prospective study. *J. Affect. Disord.*, **109,** 133–138.
71. Blumenthal, J.A., Lett, H.S., Babyak, M.A. et al. (2003) Depression as a risk factor for mortality after coronary artery bypass surgery. *Lancet*, **362,** 604–609.
72. Appels, A. and Mulder, P. (1988) Excess fatigue as a precursor of myocardial infarction. *Eur. Heart J.*, **9,** 758–764.
73. Anda, R., Williamson, D., Jones, D. et al. (1993) Depressed affect, hopelessness, and the risk of ischemic heart disease in a cohort of U.S. adults. *Epidemiology*, **4,** 285–294.
74. Aromaa, A., Raitasalo, R., Reunanen, A. et al. (1994) Depression and cardiovascular diseases. *Acta Psychiatr. Scand.*, **377** (Suppl.), 77–82.
75. Everson, S.A., Goldberg, D.E., Kaplan, G.A. et al. (1996) Hopelessness and risk of mortality and incidence of myocardial infarction and cancer. *Psychosom. Med.*, **58,** 113–121.
76. Barefoot, J.C. and Schroll, M. (1996) Symptoms of depression, acute myocardial infarction, and total mortality in a community sample. *Circulation*, **93,** 1976–1980.

77. Pratt, L.A., Ford, D.E., Crum, R.M. et al. (1996) Depression, psychotropic medication, and risk of myocardial infarction: prospective data from the Baltimore ECA follow-up. *Circulation*, **94,** 3123–3129.

78. Ariyo, A.A., Haan, M., Tangen, C.M. et al. (2000) Depressive symptoms and risks of coronary heart disease and mortality in elderly Americans. *Circulation*, **102,** 1773–1779.

79. Ferketich, A.K., Schwartzbaum, J.A., Frid, D.J. and Moeschberger, M.L. (2000) Depression as an antecedent to heart disease among women and men in the NHANES I study. National Health and Nutrition Examination Survey. *Arch. Intern. Med.*, **160,** 1261–1268.

80. Penninx F B.W., Beekman F A.T. Honig F A., et al. (2001) Depression and cardiac mortality: results from a community-based longitudinal study. *Arch. Gen. Psychiatry*, **58,** 221–227.

81. Wulsin, L., Evans, J., Vasan, R. et al. (2005) Depressive symptoms, coronary heart disease, and overall mortality in the Framingham Heart Study. *Psychosom. Med.*, **67,** 697–702.

82. Surtees, P., Wainwright, N., Luben, R. et al. (2008) Depression and ischemic heart disease mortality: evidence from the EPIC-Norfolk United Kingdom prospective cohort study. *Am. J. Psychiatry*, **165,** 515–523.

83. Kendler, K.S., Gardner, C.O., Fiske, A. and Gatz, M. (2009) Major depression and coronary artery disease in the Swedish Twin Registry. *Arch. Gen. Psychiatry*, **66,** 857–863.

84. Faris, R., Purcell, H., Henein, M. and Coats, A. (2002) Clinical depression is common and significantly associated with reduced survival in patients with non-ischaemic heart failure. *Eur. J. Heart Failure*, **4,** 541–551.

85. de Denus, S., Spinler, S., Jessup, M. and Kao, A. (2004) History of depression as a predictor of adverse outcomes in patients hospitalized for decompensated heart failure. *Pharmacotherapy*, **24,** 1306–1310.

86. Sullivan, M., Levy, W., Crane, B. et al. (2004) Usefulness of depression to predict time to combined end point of transplant or death for outpatients with advanced heart failure. *Am. J. Cardiol.*, **94,** 1577–1580.

87. Junger, J., Schellberg, D., Muller-Tasch, T. et al. (2005) Depression increasingly predicts mortality in the course of congestive heart failure. *Eur. J. Heart Failure*, **7,** 261–267.

88. Friedmann, E., Thomas, S., Liu, F. et al. (2006) Relationship of depression, anxiety, and social isolation to chronic heart failure outpatient mortality. *Am. Heart J.*, **152,** 940.e1–940.e8.

89. Jiang, W., Kuchibhatla, M., Clary, G. et al. (2007) Relationship between depressive symptoms and long-term mortality in patients with heart failure. *Am. Heart J.*, **154,** 102–108.

90. Sherwood, A., Blumenthal, J., Trivedi, R. et al. (2007) Relationship of depression to death or hospitalization in patients with heart failure. *Arch. Int. Med.*, **167,** 367–373.
91. Macchia, A., Monte, S., Pellegrini, F. et al. (2008) Depression worsens outcomes in elderly patients with heart failure: an analysis of 48,117 patients in a community setting. *Eur. J. Heart Failure*, **10,** 714–721.
92. Parissis, J., Nikolaou, M., Farmakis, D. et al. (2008) Clinical and prognostic implications of self-rating depression scales and plasma B-type natriuretic peptide in hospitalized patients with chronic heart failure. *Heart*, **94,** 585–589.
93. Albert, N., Fonarow, G., Abraham, W. et al. (2009) Depression and clinical outcomes in heart failure: an OPTIMIZE-HF analysis. *Am. J. Med.*, **122,** 366–373.
94. Schiffer, A., Pelle, A., Smith, O. et al. (2009) Somatic versus cognitive symptoms of depression as predictors of all-cause mortality and health status in chronic heart failure. *J. Clin. Psychiatry*, **70,** 1667–1673.

CHAPTER 2

The Association between Depression and Heart Disease: The Role of Biological Mechanisms

Palmiero Monteleone

Department of Psychiatry, University of Naples SUN, Naples, Italy

In the past 15 years, evidence has been provided that physically healthy subjects who suffer from depression are at increased risk for cardiovascular morbidity and mortality [1, 2], and that the occurrence of depression in patients with either unstable angina [3] or myocardial infarction (MI) [4] increases the risk for subsequent cardiac death. Moreover, epidemiological studies have proved that cardiovascular disease is a risk factor for depression, since the prevalence of depression in individuals with a recent MI or with coronary artery disease (CAD) or congestive heart failure has been found to be significantly higher than in the general population [5, 6].

These findings suggest a bidirectional association between depression and cardiovascular disease. The pathophysiological mechanisms underlying this association are, at present, largely unclear, but several candidate mechanisms have been proposed. This chapter selectively

Depression and Heart Disease Edited by Alexander Glassman, Mario Maj and Norman Sartorius
© 2011 John Wiley & Sons, Ltd

reviews recent research on biological mechanisms that may explain the association between depression and ischaemic heart disease by grouping them into four areas: autonomic nervous system dysregulation; blood clotting and endothelial dysfunctions; inflammation; neuroendocrine abnormalities.

AUTONOMIC NERVOUS SYSTEM DYSREGULATION

Autonomic nervous system dysregulation is one of the most plausible candidate mechanisms underlying the relationship between depression and ischaemic heart disease, since changes of autonomic tone have been detected in both depression and cardiovascular disease [7], and autonomic imbalance, that is reduced parasympathetic and/or increased sympathetic tone, has been found to lower the threshold for ventricular tachycardia, ventricular fibrillation and sudden cardiac death in patients with CAD [8, 9].

One of the first research findings supporting an autonomic nervous system dysregulation in depression was the report of elevated plasma and urinary noradrenaline levels in medically well, depressed patients [10–12], which suggested increased activity of the sympathetic nervous system. The increased sympathetic tone is probably responsible for the elevation of resting heart rate that has been observed in both medically well patients with major depression [13, 14] and depressed patients with CAD [15, 16]. An increased basal heart rate has been found to be predictive of enhanced morbidity and mortality related to cardiovascular disease [17].

Autonomic dysregulation may also manifest in the form of altered heart rate variability (HRV). HRV refers to beat-to-beat changes in heart rate as the heart responds to internal and external stimuli. Low HRV indicates excessive sympathetic or reduced parasympathetic heart rate modulation, and is a powerful, independent predictor of mortality in patients with CAD [18, 19]. Many, although not all, studies have reported a decreased HRV in depressed patients with or without cardiovascular disease compared with non-depressed control subjects [7, 20]. Furthermore, there seems to be a direct correlation between severity of the depressive symptomatology and reduction of HRV [21].

Low HRV has been reported to account for approximately 30% of depression-related mortality risk in patients with a recent MI [22]. The combination of HRV and heart rate turbulence was found to be a better predictor of mortality risk in those patients. Heart rate turbulence analysis quantifies the heart rate response to premature ventricular contractions and represents a further method to assess autonomic nervous system function. Normally, after a premature ventricular contraction, heart rate first accelerates and then decelerates. A heart rate response to premature ventricular contractions differing from this pattern was associated with a greater risk of mortality in post-MI depressed patients [22] and the combination of heart rate turbulence and HRV was found to explain about half of the depression-related mortality risk in those patients.

Further indexes of the autonomic nervous system modulation of cardiovascular functions are the heart rate response to stressors, the baroreflex function and the ventricular repolarisation as expressed by the QT interval variability. Evidence has been provided that depression is associated with significant dysregulations of all these measures.

Abnormally increased heart rate responses to both physical and psychological stressors have been detected in medically well subjects with major depression [23, 24], and depressed patients with CAD have been shown to exhibit increased heart rate response to orthostatic challenge compared with non-depressed individuals with CAD [25].

A reduction in baroreflex sensitivity has been found to increase the risk of death in patients recovering from MI [26], and depression has been found to be associated with a reduction in baroreflex sensitivity in patients with CAD [27]. Another study [28] did not confirm this association in a sample of post-MI patients, but almost 80% of those patients were taking beta-blockers. One more study [29] found a reduced baroreflex function in post-MI depressed patients, but not in those receiving beta-blockers.

The QT interval variability reflects beat-to-beat fluctuations of ventricular repolarisation time, and increased QT variability has been associated with an increased risk of arrhythmias and sudden cardiac death [30, 31]. In the only study performed so far [32], post-MI depressed patients were found to have increased QT variability, especially in the morning hours (6:00 a.m.), when the risk of sudden cardiac death has been found to be maximum [33].

BLOOD CLOTTING AND ENDOTHELIAL DYSFUNCTION

Imbalance between prothrombotic and antithrombotic mechanisms and endothelial dysfunction have been suggested to contribute to the increased risk of cardiac events in both medically well patients with depression and depressed patients with CAD.

Depression has been consistently associated with enhanced platelet activation, as reflected by increased 5-HT2 receptor binding sites on the platelet surface [34, 35] and increased serotonin-induced platelet calcium mobilisation [36] in depressed patients compared with healthy control subjects. Since serotonin secreted by platelets after their activation induces platelet aggregation and coronary vasoconstriction through the stimulation of 5-HT2 receptors [37], these findings support the notion of a dysfunction of serotonin-mediated platelet aggregation in patients with depression, which may have prothrombotic effects. Moreover, increased plasma levels of pro-thrombogenic factors such as platelet-factor-4 (PF-4), β-thromboglobulin, platelet-endothelial cell adhesion molecule-1 and thromboxane have been reported in depressed patients with acute CAD [38]. On the other hand, evidence has accumulated that selective serotonin reuptake inhibitors (SSRIs) reduce platelet hyperreactivity and hyperaggregation of depressed patients [39, 40] and reduce the release of the platelet/endothelial biomarkers β-thromboglobulin, P-selectin and E-selectin in depressed patients with acute CAD [41]. This may explain the efficacy of SSRIs in reducing the risk of mortality in depressed patients with CAD [42–44].

Further evidence of the association between depression and pro-thrombotic mechanisms has been provided by the finding of enhanced levels of the soluble CD40 ligand in drug-naïve patients with a first major depressive episode [45]. The CD40 ligand is a transmembrane protein rapidly released from platelets upon their activation, which elicits pro-inflammatory and prothrombotic activities favouring and accelerating the progression of atherosclerosis [46]. Moreover, Leo et al. [45] found that, in drug-naïve major depressive patients, soluble CD40 ligand levels were positively correlated with those of the procoagulative factors FVIIa and F1 + 2 and the pro-inflammatory markers interleukin (IL)-6, IL-1 and tumour necrosis factor (TNF)-α. This suggests that the CD40 ligand released from activated platelets may induce procoagulative and pro-inflammatory responses, in major depressive patients, which in turn may favour ischaemic events. However, circulating levels of the soluble CD40 ligand have been found to be not significantly different between depressed and non-depressed patients with recent MI [47].

There is also growing evidence for endothelial dysfunction as a potential link between depression and ischaemic heart disease. In support of this hypothesis, several studies have shown that reduced endothelium-dependent flow-mediated vasodilatation assessed by brachial artery ultrasound occurs in depressed adults with or without CAD [48–50]. This was observed not only in older depressed individuals, who could have an underlying atherosclerosis contributing to the endothelial dysfunction, but also in adolescent women who were too young to have developed significant atherosclerosis [51]. Furthermore, circulating levels of the soluble intercellular adhesion molecule, which is a marker of endothelial activation, have been reported to be significantly higher in depressed patients who had recently experienced an acute coronary event than in non-depressed ones [52].

Decreased nitric oxide (NO) production has been suggested to contribute to the increased platelet reactivity and reduced endothelium-dependent vasodilatation of depressed patients and, therefore, to the increased risk of cardiovascular disease in patients with major depression. NO is not only responsible for vasodilatation, but also inhibits platelet aggregation and adhesion. It is synthesised from L-arginine by the enzyme nitric oxidase synthase (NOS), which exists in different isoforms. The endothelial isoform (eNOS) is present in both the endothelium and platelets, and both endothelium-derived and platelet-derived NO play a role in preventing platelet adhesion to the vascular wall and platelet aggregation [53], therefore inhibiting the thrombus formation, which has a major role in triggering coronary accidents. Recently, platelet NOS activity and plasma levels of nitrogen dioxides, metabolites of NO, have been found dramatically decreased in patients with major depression [54], whereas the administration of the SSRI paroxetine has found to be associated with a significant increase of platelet eNOS activity in major depressive patients [55], which may explain the cardiovascular protective effect of this drug in depressed patients with CAD.

INFLAMMATION

Atherosclerosis with subsequent plaque rupture and thrombosis is the main determinant of ischaemic cardiovascular events, and atherosclerosis itself is now recognised to be fundamentally an inflammatory disease [56]. Since activation of inflammatory processes is common to both depression and cardiovascular disease, it would be reasonable to argue that the link between depression and ischaemic heart disease might be mediated by inflammation.

Evidence has been provided that major depression is associated with a significant increase in circulating levels of both pro-inflammatory cytokines, such as IL-6 and TNF-α, and inflammatory acute phase proteins, especially the C-reactive protein (CRP) [57, 58], and that antidepressant treatment is able to normalise CRP levels irrespective of whether or not patients are clinically improved [59]. Furthermore, the acute phase proteins, CRP and serum amyloid A have been found to be significantly elevated also in remitted depressed patients [60]. These findings, taken together, support the idea that patients with major depression have a pro-inflammatory profile even when they are euthymic, and that antidepressants are able to suppress this profile.

It has been proposed that depression promotes weight accumulation, especially in the form of visceral fat, which in turn activates an inflammatory response through two possible mechanisms: the release of the fat-derived IL-6, which stimulates the liver production of CRP; and the synthesis of the fat-derived hormone leptin, which activates the production of IL-6 from white blood cells and/or vascular endothelial cells with the subsequent stimulation of liver CRP synthesis [61]. Conversely, an excessive production of the pro-inflammatory cytokines IL-1 and TNF-α and of IL-2 has been suggested to contribute to the pathophysiology of depression [62] and several studies have provided the evidence not only of enhanced levels of those cytokines in patients with major depression [63–65], but also of depressive symptom induction by the exogenous administration of TNF-α and α-interferon in humans [66, 67]. Furthermore, the activation of the hypothalamic-pituitary-adrenal (HPA) axis occurring in depression [68–70] may result in the release of pro-inflammatory cytokines, which in turn are able to stimulate the HPA axis [71], thus perpetuating a vicious circle which favours atherogenic and pro-ischaemic processes.

Activation of the inflammatory system is also linked to ischaemic cardiovascular events in people with CAD. A recent meta-analysis has shown that CRP has a significant role in predicting recurrent MI and cardiac death [72] and that the combined presence of elevated CRP, IL-6 and TNF-α was associated with elevated risk of clinical manifestations of CAD [73]. Recent studies exploring inflammatory markers in CAD patients with or without major depression have provided mixed results. In patients with a past history of acute coronary syndrome, the severity of depression was positively correlated with CRP levels, but not with IL-6 or TNF-α concentrations [74], while higher levels of CRP were detected in depressed CAD patients not using statins, but not in those treated with these drugs [52]. In patients with recent MI or in subjects after coronary revascularisation, no difference was found between those with major depression and those without depression in circulating levels of several inflammatory markers [75, 76]. However, most of the participants were taking statins and this could have affected the results. In addition, two recent studies even reported reduced levels of CRP, fibrinogen, IL-6 and ferritin in depressed compared with non-depressed individuals with stable CAD [77, 78]. Finally, Vaccarino et al. [79] assessed specifically whether inflammation is the mechanism linking depression to ischaemic cardiac events and found that, in women with suspected coronary ischaemia, depression was associated with increased circulating levels of CRP and IL-6 and was a strong predictor of ischaemic cardiac events, but the two inflammatory biomarkers explained only a small portion of the association between depression and ischaemic heart events.

Pro-inflammatory cytokines also affect both central and peripheral serotonergic systems. It has been reported that IL-1 and α-interferon induce the enzyme indole-amine-2,3 di-oxygenase, which converts tryptophan into quinurenine, leading to a depletion of the peripheral amino acid, with a consequent decrease in its availability for brain serotonin synthesis. These processes would facilitate the development of depressive symptoms, on the one hand, and, on the other, platelet aggregation, fibrinolysis and occlusion of coronary arteries [80].

It has been hypothesised that alterations in polyunsatured fatty acids (PUFAs) are also involved in the connection between depression, inflammation and CAD. Indeed, omega-3 PUFAs decrease circulating markers of inflammation and endothelial dysfunction [81] and reduce CAD mortality, especially sudden cardiac death [82]. Depression has been found to be associated with decreased levels of omega-3 PUFA [83] and increased concentrations of homocysteine [84], which represents an independent risk factor for the development of atherosclerosis. Furthermore, CAD patients with depression have lower plasma concentrations of omega-3 PUFA and a greater imbalance between omega-3 (anti-inflammatory) and omega-6 (pro-inflammatory) PUFA than patients without depression [85].

NEUROENDOCRINE ABNORMALITIES

Major depression has been consistently associated with hyperactivity of the HPA axis, with a consequent overstimulation of the sympathetic nervous system, which in turn results in increased circulating catecholamine levels and enhanced serum cortisol concentrations [68–70]. This may cause an imbalance in sympathetic and parasympathetic activity, which results in elevated heart rate and blood pressure, reduced HRV, disruption of ventricular electrophysiology with increased risk of ventricular arrhythmias as well as an increased risk of atherosclerotic plaque rupture and acute coronary thrombosis. Moreover, increased plasma levels of catecholamines may promote platelet activation either directly or indirectly by inhibiting the synthesis of protective vascular endothelial eicosanoids and increasing the release of platelet-derived growth factor. Platelet activation, in turn, may promote damage to vascular endothelium and the formation of atherosclerotic plaques through the release of PF-4, β-thromboglobulin, thromboxane A2 and the platelet activating factor [86].

Hypercortisolaemia also plays a role in the distribution of body fat, increasing the stores of intra-abdominal fat, which is a well-known risk factor for CAD. Visceral fat has been found two times higher in depressed women than in healthy control subjects [87] and, as suggested above [61], it could be responsible for increased production of pro-inflammatory cytokines. In addition, glucocorticoids mobilise free fatty acids, causing endothelial inflammation and excessive clotting, and are associated with hypertension, hypercholesterolaemia and glucose dysregulation [88, 89], which are risk factors for CAD. Increased circulating lipids and endothelial shearing stress can lead to vascular damage and plaque formation [90].

CONCLUSIONS

Although all the above-described biological mechanisms have been demonstrated to represent independent risk factors for both cardio-vascular disease in physically healthy depressed individuals and ischaemic events in CAD patients with or without depression, it is not surprising that several interactions exist among them (Figure 2.1). As a matter of fact, evidence has been provided that a cholinergic vagal efferent pathway inhibits pro-inflammatory cytokine release [91], so it is plausible that the depression-induced autonomic nervous system imbalance, with increased sympathetic and/or decreased parasympathetic tone, may lead, on the one hand, to low HRV and other cardiac electrophysiological alterations and, on the other, to activation of inflammatory processes. In support of this idea, inverse correlations between HRV and some inflammatory markers have been found in depressed patients with CAD [92] as well as in healthy subjects and non-depressed patients with acute or stable CAD [93]. On the other hand, inflammation may induce endothelial dysfunction through CRP-induced decrease in eNOS activity and subsequent reduction in NO synthesis [94], and may activate the HPA axis, perpetuating depression-induced hypercortisolaemia, which may result in further increase in inflammation through enhanced synthesis of IL-6 by increased visceral fat stores. Moreover, increased plasma levels of catecholamines resulting from activation of the sympathetic nervous system may promote platelet activation and precipitate

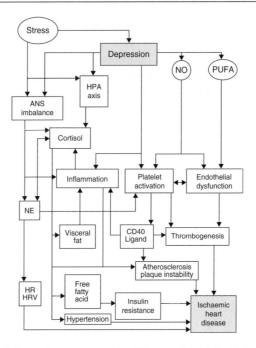

Figure 2.1 Schematic representation of the possible biological connections between depression and ischaemic heart disease. ANS – autonomic nervous system; HPA – hypothalamic-pituitary-adrenal axis; HR – heart rate; HRV – heart rate variability; NE – noradrenaline; NO – nitric oxide; PUFA – polyunsatured fatty acids.

thrombotic events. Autonomic dysfunction, HPA activation and inflammation may also account for the deleterious effects of stress on the cardiovascular system [84] and it is well known that stress in daily life may influence the onset and course of depression [83].

In conclusion, several biological pathways may underlie the association between depression and ischaemic heart disease. In the future, it may be expected that genetic studies will substantially contribute to the progress of knowledge in this area, since the recognition of a genetic predisposition to any of the above-mentioned biological mechanisms may lead to the identification of pathogenetic pathways common to both depression and CAD.

REFERENCES

1. Glassman, A.H. and Shapiro, P.A. (1998) Depression and the course of coronary artery disease. *Am. J. Psychiatry*, **155,** 4–11.
2. Musselman, D.L., Evans, D.L. and Nemeroff, C.B. (1998) The relationship of depression to cardiovascular disease: epidemiology, biology, and treatment. *Arch. Gen. Psychiatry*, **55,** 580–592.
3. Lesperance, F., Juneau, M. and Theroux, P. (2000) Depression and 1-year prognosis in unstable angina. *Arch. Intern. Med.*, **160,** 1354–1360.
4. Lespérance, F., Frasure-Smith, N., Talajic, M. and Bourassa, M.G. (2002) Five-year risk of cardiac mortality in relation to initial severity and 1-year changes in depression symptoms after myocardial infarction. *Circulation*, **105,** 1049–1053.
5. Schleifer, S.J., Macari-Hinson, M.M., Coyle, D.A. et al. (1989) The nature and course of depression following myocardial infarction. *Arch. Int. Med.*, **149,** 1785–1789.
6. Freedland, K.E., Miller, G.E. and Sheps, D.S. (2006) The great debate, revisited. *Psychosom. Med.*, **68,** 179–184.
7. Carney, R.M. and Freedland, K.E. (2009) Depression and heart rate variability in patients with coronary heart disease. *Cleve. Clin. J. Med.*, **76** (Suppl. 2), S13–S17.
8. Schwartz, P.J. and Vanoli, E. (1981) Cardiac arrhythmias elicited by interaction between acute myocardial ischemia and sympathetic hyperactivity: a new experimental model for the study of antiarrhythmic drugs. *J. Cardiovasc. Pharmacol.*, **3,** 1251–1259.
9. Podrid, P.J., Fuchs, T. and Candinas, R. (1990) Role of the sympathetic nervous system in the genesis of ventricular arrhythmia. *Circulation*, **82** (Suppl. 2), I103–I113.
10. Esler, M., Turbott, J., Schwarz, R. et al. (1982) The peripheral kinetics of norepinephrine in depressive illness. *Arch. Gen. Psychiatry*, **39,** 295–300.
11. Roy, A., Pickar, D., De Jong, J. et al. (1988) Norepinephrine and its metabolites in cerebrospinal fluid, plasma, and urine. Relationship to hypothalamic-pituitary-adrenal axis function in depression. *Arch. Gen. Psychiatry*, **45,** 849–857.
12. Veith, R.C., Lewis, N., Linares, O.A. et al. (1994) Sympathetic nervous system activity in major depression: basal and desipramine-induced alterations in plasma norepinephrine kinetics. *Arch. Gen. Psychiatry*, **51,** 411–422.
13. Forbes, L.M. and Chaney, R.H. (1980) Cardiovascular changes during acute depression. *Psychosomatics*, **21,** 472–477.

14. Lahmeyer, H.W. and Bellur, S.N. (1987) Cardiac regulation and depression. *J. Psychiatr. Res.*, **21**, 1–6.

15. Carney, R.M., Rich, M.W., teVelde, A. et al. (1988) The relationship between heart rate, heart rate variability and depression in patients with coronary artery disease. *J. Psychosom. Res.*, **32**, 159–164.

16. Carney, R.M., Freedland, K.E., Veith, R.C. et al. (1999) Major depression, heart rate, and plasma norepinephrine in patients with coronary heart disease. *Biol. Psychiatry*, **45**, 458–463.

17. Ferrari, R., Censi, S., Mastrorilli, F. and Boraso, A. (2003) Prognostic benefits of heart rate reduction in cardiovascular disease. *Eur. Heart J.*, **5** (Suppl. G), G10–G14.

18. Kleiger, R.E., Miller, J.P., Bigger, J.T. and Moss, A.J. (1987) Decreased heart rate variability and its association with increased mortality after acute myocardial infarction. *Am. J. Cardiol.*, **59**, 256–262.

19. Tapanainen, J.M., Thomsem, P.E.B., Køber, L. et al. (2002) Fractal analysis of heart rate variability and mortality after an acute myocardial infarction. *Am. J. Cardiol.*, **90**, 347–352.

20. Gehi, A., Mangano, D., Pipkin, S. et al. (2005) Depression and heart rate variability in patients with stable coronary heart disease: findings from the Heart and Soul Study. *Arch. Gen. Psychiatry*, **62**, 661–666.

21. Krittayaphong, R., Cascio, W.E., Light, K.C. et al. (1997) Heart rate variability in patients with coronary artery disease: differences in patients with higher and lower depression scores. *Psychosom. Med.*, **59**, 231–235.

22. Carney, R.M., Blumenthal, J.A., Freedland, K.E. et al. (2005) Low heart rate variability and the effect of depression on post-myocardial infarction mortality. *Arch. Intern. Med.*, **165**, 1486–1491.

23. Gotthardt, U., Schweiger, U., Fahrenberg, J. et al. (1995) Cortisol, ACTH, and cardiovascular response to a cognitive challenge paradigm in aging and depression. *Am. J. Physiol.*, **268**, 865–873.

24. Lehofer, M., Moser, M., Hoehn-Saric, R. et al. (1997) Major depression and cardiac autonomic control. *Biol. Psychiatry*, **42**, 914–919.

25. Carney, R.M., Freedland, K.E., Veith, R.C. et al. (1999) Major depression, heart rate, and plasma norepinephrine in patients with coronary heart disease. *Biol. Psychiatry*, **45**, 458–463.

26. Mortara, A., La Rovere, M.T., Pinna, G.D. et al. (1997) Arterial baroreflex modulation of heart rate in chronic heart failure: clinical and hemodynamic correlates and prognostic implications. *Circulation*, **96**, 3450–3458.

27. Watkins, L.L. and Grossman, P. (1999) Association of depressive symptoms with reduced baroreflex cardiac control in coronary artery disease. *Am. Heart J.*, **137**, 453–457.

28. Watkins, L.L., Blumenthal, J.A. and Carney, R.M. (2002) Association of anxiety with reduced baroreflex cardiac control in patients after acute myocardial infarction. *Am. Heart J.*, **143**, 460–466.

29. Pitzalis, M.V., Iacoviello, M., Todarello, O. et al. (2001) Depression but not anxiety influences the autonomic control of heart rate after myocardial infarction. *Am. Heart J.*, **141**, 765–771.

30. Atiga, W.L., Calkins, H., Lawrence, J.H. et al. (1998) Beat-to-beat repolarization lability identifies patients at risk for sudden cardiac death. *J. Cardiovasc. Electrophysiol.*, **9**, 899–908.

31. Maison-Blanche, P. and Coumel, P. (1997) Changes in repolarization dynamicity and the assessment of arrhythmic risk. *Pacing Clin. Electrophysiol.*, **20**, 2614–2624.

32. Carney, R.M., Freedland, K.E., Stein, P.K. et al. (2003) Effects of depression on QT interval variability after myocardial infarction. *Psychosom. Med.*, **65**, 177–180.

33. Muller, J.E., Ludmer, P.L., Willich, S.N. et al. (1987) Circadian variation in the frequency of sudden cardiac death. *Circulation*, **75**, 131–138.

34. Hrdina, P.D., Bakish, D., Ravindran, A. et al. (1997) Platelet serotonergic indices in major depression: up-regulation of 5-HT2A receptors unchanged by antidepressant treatment. *Psychiatr. Res.*, **66**, 73–85.

35. Serres, F., Azorin, J.M., Valli, M. and Jeanningros, R. (1999) Evidence for an increase in functional platelet 5-HT2A receptors in depressed patients using the new ligand [125I]-DOI. *Eur. Psychiatry*, **14**, 451–457.

36. Delisi, J.S., Konopka, L.M., Russell, K. et al. (1999) Platelet cytosolic calcium hyperresponsivity to serotonin in patients with hypertension and depressive symptoms. *Biol. Psychiatry*, **45**, 1035–1042.

37. Hrdina, P.D., Bakish, D., Chudzik, J. et al. (1995) Serotonergic markers in platelets of patients with major depression: upregulation of 5-HT2 receptors. *J. Psychiatry Neurosci.*, **20**, 11–19.

38. Serebruany, V.L., Glassman, A.H., Malinin, A.I. et al. (2003) Enhanced platelet/endothelial activation in depressed patients with acute coronary syndromes: evidence from recent clinical trials. *Blood Coagul. Fibrinolysis*, **14**, 563–567.

39. Musselman, D.L., Marzec, U.M., Manatunga, A. et al. (2000) Platelet reactivity in depressed patients treated with paroxetine: preliminary findings. *Arch. Gen. Psychiatry*, **57**, 875–882.

40. Serebruany, V.L., Gurbel, P.A. and O'Connor, C.M. (2001) Platelet inhibition by sertraline and *N*-desmethylsertraline: a possible missing link between depression, coronary events, and mortality benefits of selective serotonin reuptake inhibitors. *Pharm. Res.*, **43**, 453–462.

41. Serebruany, V.L., Glassman, A.H., Malinin, A.I. et al. (2003) Platelet/endothelial biomarkers in depressed patients treated with the selective serotonin reuptake inhibitor sertraline after acute coronary events: the Sertraline Antidepressant Heart Attack Randomized Trial (SADHART) platelet substudy. *Circulation*, **108**, 939–944.

42. Shapiro, P.A., Lespérance, F., Frasure-Smith, N. et al. (1999) An open-label preliminary trial of sertraline for treatment of major depression after acute myocardial infarction (the SADHART trial): Sertraline Anti-Depressant Heart Attack Trial. *Am. Heart J.*, **137**, 1100–1106.

43. Sauer, W.H., Berlin, J.A. and Kimmel, S.E. (2001) Selective serotonin reuptake inhibitors and myocardial infarction. *Circulation*, **104**, 1894–1898.

44. Glassman, A.H., O'Connor, C.M., Califf, R.M. et al. (2002) Sertraline treatment of major depression in patients with acute MI or unstable angina. *JAMA*, **288**, 701–709.

45. Leo, R., Di Lorenzo, G., Tesauro, M. et al. (2006) Association between enhanced soluble CD40 ligand and proinflammatory and prothrombotic states in major depressive disorder: pilot observations on the effects of selective serotonin reuptake inhibitor therapy. *J. Clin. Psychiatry*, **67**, 1760–1766.

46. André, P., Nannizzi-Alaimo, L., Prasad, S.K. and Phillips, D.R. (2002) Platelet-derived CD40L: the switch-hitting player of cardiovascular disease. *Circulation*, **106**, 896–899.

47. Schins, A., Hamulyák, K., Scharpé, S. et al. (2004) Whole blood serotonin and platelet activation in depressed post-myocardial infarction patients. *Life Sci.*, **76**, 637–650.

48. Broadley, A.J., Korszun, A., Jones, C.J. and Frenneaux, M.P. (2002) Arterial endothelial function is impaired in treated depression. *Heart*, **88**, 521–523.

49. Sherwood, A., Hinderliter, A.L., Watkins, L.L. et al. (2005) Impaired endothelial function in coronary heart disease patients with depressive symptomatology. *J. Am. Coll. Cardiol.*, **46**, 656–659.

50. Wagner, J.A., Tennen, H., Mansoor, G.A. and Abbott, G. (2006) History of major depressive disorder and endothelial function in postmenopausal women. *Psychosom. Med.*, **68**, 80–86.

51. Tomfohr, L.M., Martin, T.M. and Miller, G.E. (2008) Symptoms of depression and impaired endothelial function in healthy adolescent women. *J. Behav. Med.*, **31**, 137–143.

52. Lesperance, F., Frasure-Smith, N., Theroux, P. and Irwin, M. (2004) The association between major depression and levels of soluble inter-cellular adhesion molecule 1, interleukin-6, and C-reactive protein in

patients with recent acute coronary syndromes. *Am. J. Psychiatry*, **161**, 271–277.

53. Freedman, J.E., Loscalzo, J., Barnard, M.R. et al. (1997) Nitric oxide released from activated platelets inhibits platelet recruitment. *J. Clin. Invest.*, **100**, 350–356.

54. Chrapko, W.E., Jurasz, P., Radomski, M.W. et al. (2004) Decreased nitric oxide synthase and plasma nitric oxide metabolites in major depressive disorder. *Biol. Psychiatry*, **56**, 129–134.

55. Chrapko, W., Jurasz, P., Radomski, M.W. et al. (2006) Alteration of decreased plasma NO metabolites and platelet NO synthase activity by paroxetine in depressed patients. *Neuropsychopharmacology*, **31**, 1286–1293.

56. Ross, R. (1999) Atherosclerosis: an inflammatory disease. *N. Engl. J. Med.*, **340**, 115–126.

57. Maes, M., Meltzer, H.Y., Bosmans, E. et al. (1995) Increased plasma concentrations of interleukin-6, soluble interleukin-6, soluble interleukin-2 and transferring receptor in major depression. *J. Affect Disord.*, **34**, 301–309.

58. Maes, M., Bosmans, E., De Jongh, R. et al. (1997) Increased serum IL-6 and IL-1 receptor antagonist concentrations in major depression and treatment resistant depression. *Cytokine*, **9**, 853–858.

59. O'Brien, S., Scott, L.V. and Dinan, T.G. (2006) Antidepressant therapy and C-reactive protein levels. *Br. J. Psychiatry*, **188**, 449–452.

60. Kling, M.A., Alesci, S., Csako, G. et al. (2007) Sustained low-grade proinflammatory state in unmedicated remitted women with major depressive disorder as evidenced by elevated serum levels of the acute phase proteins C-reactive protein and serum amyloid A. *Biol. Psychiatry*, **62**, 309–313.

61. Miller, G.E., Freedland, K.E., Carney, R.M. et al. (2003) Pathways linking depression, adiposity, and inflammatory markers in healthy young adults. *Brain Behav. Immun.*, **17**, 276–285.

62. Smith, R.S. (1991) The macrophage theory of depression. *Med. Hypotheses*, **35**, 298–306.

63. Maes, M. (1995) Evidence for an immune response in major depression: a review and hypothesis. *Prog. Neuropsychopharmacol. Biol. Psychiatry*, **19**, 11–38.

64. Miller, G.E., Stetler, C.A., Carney, R.M. et al. (2002) Clinical depression and inflammatory risk markers for coronary heart disease. *Am. J. Cardiol.*, **90**, 1279–1283.

65. Dantzer, R. (2006) Cytokine, sickness behavior, and depression. *Neurol. Clin.*, **24**, 441–460.

66. Niiranen, A., Laaksonen, R., Iivanainen, M. et al. (1988) Behavioral assessment of patients treated with alpha-interferon. *Acta Psychiatr. Scand.*, **78**, 622–626.

67. Spriggs, D.R., Sherman, M.L., Michie, H. et al. (1988) Recombinant human tumor necrosis factor administered as a 24-hour intravenous infusion. A phase1 and pharmacology study. *J. Natl. Cancer Inst.*, **80**, 1039–1044.

68. Carroll, B.J., Feinberg, M., Greden, J.F. et al. (1981) A specific laboratory test for the diagnosis of melancholia. Standardization, validation and clinical utility. *Arch. Gen. Psychiatry*, **38**, 15–22.

69. Banki, C.M., Karmacsi, L., Bassette, G. and Nemeroff, C.B. (1992) CSF corticotropin releasing and somatostatin in major depression: response to antidepressant treatment and relapse. *Eur. Neuropsychopharmacol.*, **2**, 107–113.

70. Musselman, D.L. and Nemeroff, C.B. (1996) Depression and endocrine disorders: focus on the thyroid and adrenal system. *Br. J. Psychiatry*, **30** (Suppl.), 123–128.

71. Cassidy, E.M. and O'Keane, V. (2000) Depression and interferon-alpha therapy. *Br. J. Psychiatry*, **176**, 494.

72. Danesh, J., Wheeler, J.G., Hirschfield, G.M. et al. (2004) C-reactive protein and other circulating markers of inflammation in the prediction of coronary heart disease. *N. Engl. J. Med.*, **350**, 1387–1397.

73. Cesari, M., Penninx, B.W., Newman, A.B. et al. (2003) Inflammatory markers and onset of cardiovascular events: results from the Health ABC study. *Circulation*, **108**, 2317–2322.

74. Miller, G.E., Freedland, K.E., Duntley, S. and Carney, R.M. (2005) Relation of depressive symptoms to C-reactive protein and pathogen burden (cytomegalovirus, herpes simplex virus, Epstein-Barr virus) in patients with earlier acute coronary syndromes. *Am. J. Cardiol.*, **95**, 317–321.

75. Janszky, I., Lekander, M., Blom, M. et al. (2005) Self-rated health and vital exhaustion, but not depression, is related to inflammation in women with coronary heart disease. *Brain Behav. Immun.*, **19**, 555–563.

76. Schins, A., Tulner, D., Lousberg, R. et al. (2005) Inflammatory markers in depressed post-myocardial infarction patients. *J. Psychiatr. Res.*, **39**, 137–144.

77. Whooley, M.A., Caska, C.M., Hendrickson, B.E. et al. (2007) Depression and inflammation in patients with coronary heart disease: findings from the Heart and Soul Study. *Biol. Psychiatry*, **62**, 314–320.

78. Baune, B.T., Neuhaser, H., Ellert, U. and Berger, K. (2010) The role of the inflammatory markers ferritin, transferrin and fibrinogen in the

relationship between major depression and cardiovascular disorders – The German Health Interview and Examination Survey. *Acta Psychiatr. Scand.*, **121**, 135–141.

79. Vaccarino, V., Johnson, D.B., Sheps, D.S. et al. (2007) Depression, inflammation, and incident cardiovascular disease in women with suspected coronary ischemia. *J. Am. Coll. Cardiol.*, **50**, 2044–2050.

80. Maes, M. (1999) Major depression and activation of the inflammatory response system, in *Cytokines, Stress and Depression* (eds R. Dantzer, E.E. Wollmann and R. Yirmiya), Kluwer, New York, pp. 25–46.

81. Hjerkinn, E.M., Seljeflot, I., Ellingsen, I. et al. (2005) Influence of long-term intervention with dietary counseling, long-chain n-3 fatty acid supplements, or both on circulating markers of endothelial activation in men with long-standing hyperlipidemia. *Am. J. Clin. Nutr.*, **81**, 583–589.

82. Kris-Etherton, P.M., Harris, W.S. and Appel, L.J. (2002) American Heart Association Nutrition Committee. Fish consumption, fish oil, omega-3 fatty acids, and cardiovascular disease. *Circulation*, **106**, 2747–2757.

83. Carney, R.M., Freedland, K.E., Rich, M.W. and Jaffe, A.S. (1995) Depression as a risk factor for cardiac events in established coronary heart disease: a review of possible mechanisms. *Ann. Behav. Med.*, **17**, 142–149.

84. Severus, W.E., Littman, A.B. and Stoll, A.L. (2001) Omega-3 fatty acids, homocysteine, and the increased risk of cardiovascular mortality in major depressive disorder. *Harv. Rev. Psychiatry*, **9**, 280–293.

85. Frasure-Smith, N., Lesperance, F. and Julien, P. (2004) Major depression is associated with lower omega-3 fatty acid levels in patients with recent acute coronary syndromes. *Biol. Psychiatry*, **55**, 891–896.

86. Musselman, D.L., Evans, D.L. and Nemeroff, C.B. (1998) The relationship of depression to cardiovascular disease. *Arch. Gen. Psychiatry*, **55**, 580–592.

87. Thakore, J.H., Richards, P.J., Reznek, R.H. et al. (1997) Increased intra–abdominal fat depression in patients with major depressive illness as measured by computed tomography. *Biol. Psychiatry*, **41**, 1140–1142.

88. Gold, P.W. and Chrousos, G.P. (1999) The endocrinology of melancholic and atypical depression: relation to neurocircuitry and somatic consequences. *Proc. Assoc. Am. Physicians*, **111**, 22–34.

89. Malhotra, S., Tesar, G.E. and Franco, K. (2000) The relationship between depression and cardiovascular disorders. *Curr. Psychiatry Rep.*, **2**, 241–246.

90. Anfossi, G. and Trovati, M. (1996) Role of catecholamines in platelet function: pathophysiological and clinical significance. *Eur. J. Clin. Invest.*, **26**, 353–370.

91. Pavlov, V.A. and Tracey, K.J. (2005) The cholinergic anti-inflammatory pathway. *Brain Behav. Immun.*, **19**, 493–499.
92. Carney, R.M., Freedland, K.E., Stein, P.K. et al. (2007) Heart rate variability and markers of inflammation and coagulation in depressed patients with coronary heart disease. *J. Psychosom. Res.*, **62**, 463–467.
93. Haensel, A., Mills, P.J., Nelesen, R.A. et al. (2008) The relationship between heart rate variability and inflammatory markers in cardiovascular diseases. *Psychoneuroendocrinology*, **33**, 1305–1312.
94. Verma, S., Wang, C.H., Li, S.H. et al. (2002) A self-fulfilling prophecy: C-reactive protein attenuates nitric oxide production and inhibits angiogenesis. *Circulation*, **106**, 913–919.

CHAPTER 3

The Association between Depression and Heart Disease: The Role of Genetic Factors

Eco de Geus

*Department of Biological Psychology,
VU University, Amsterdam, The Netherlands*

The comorbidity between major depressive disorder (MDD) and coronary artery disease (CAD) has been robustly supported by a large number of observational studies. A large meta-analysis showed MDD to be associated with an 80% increased risk of developing CAD or dying from it, although this estimate may still need to be adjusted in view of evident publication bias and incomplete and non-systematic adjustment for conventional risk factors and severity of CAD at baseline [1].

Most of the literature on this comorbidity has tended to favour the hypothesis of a causal effect of MDD on CAD, but reversed causality has also been suggested to contribute. Patients with severe CAD at baseline, and consequently a worse prognosis, may simply be more prone to report mood disturbances than less severely ill patients. Furthermore, in pre-morbid populations, insipid atherosclerosis in cerebral vessels may cause depressive symptoms before the onset of

Depression and Heart Disease Edited by Alexander Glassman, Mario Maj and Norman Sartorius
© 2011 John Wiley & Sons, Ltd

actual cardiac or cerebrovascular events, a variant of reverse causality known as the 'vascular depression' hypothesis [2].

To resolve causality, comorbidity between MDD and CAD has been addressed in longitudinal designs. Most prospective studies reported that clinical depression or depressive symptoms at baseline predicted higher incidence of heart disease at follow-up [1], which seems to favour the hypothesis of causal effects of MDD. We need to remind ourselves, however, that prediction is nothing more than an association, in this case an association of MDD at wave 1 with CAD at wave 2 of data collection. Prospective associations do not necessarily equate causation. Higher incidence of CAD in depressed individuals may reflect the operation of common underlying factors on MDD and CAD that become manifest in mental health at an earlier stage than in cardiac health. This would give rise to a prospective link between depressive symptoms and CAD, but causal effects would flow forth from the underlying factors only, explaining why behavioural or pharmacological interventions on MDD do not necessarily result in improved CAD outcomes [3, 4].

These 'third factors' may consist of environmental influences, such as early childhood trauma, low socio-economic status and poor social support networks, that affect both MDD and CAD risk. Alternatively, the association between MDD and CAD may be due to underlying genetic factors that lead to increased symptoms of anxiety and depression, but may also independently influence the atherosclerotic process. This phenomenon, where low-level biological variation has effects on multiple complex traits at the organ and behavioural level, is called genetic 'pleiotropy'. If present in a time-lagged form, that is if genetic effects on MDD risk precede effects of the same genetic variants on CAD risk, this phenomenon can cause longitudinal correlations that mimic a causal effect of MDD.

Anticipating a hypothesis in a later section of this chapter, let me illustrate genetic pleiotropy with an example. Suppose that individual differences in the responsivity of pro-inflammatory cytokines to external pathogens are governed by variants in the genes coding for these cytokines or their receptors. Further assume that increased cytokine activity has an impact on atherosclerotic processes [5, 6] as well as on mood regulation [7]. In this case, individuals with the genetic variants that cause an increased pro-inflammatory state may be at increased risk for mood disturbances through the central nervous system effect of the cytokines and at increased risk for atherosclerosis through their peripheral inflammatory effects. There is no need to assume a direct effect of mood disturbance on atherosclerosis; the double role of cytokines in the brain and the circulation simply reflects natural selection of a successful cell-to-cell signalling system that is re-employed in multiple organ systems.

A core prediction of the genetic pleiotropy hypothesis is that both depression and cardiovascular disease are heritable traits, and that part of the genetic variants causing heritability in one trait also influence the other trait. Genetically informative designs are needed to test for heritability and the presence of such underlying genetic 'third factors'. One such a design is the twin study.

TWIN STUDIES

Monozygotic (MZ) twinning occurs when, for reasons that are still incompletely understood, a fertilised egg divides before it nestles in the uterus. MZ twins inherit identical genetic material, with a few rare exceptions [8]. If more than one egg is released from the ovaries during a menstrual cycle and each egg is fertilised by a separate sperm, the result is a set of non-identical twins, also known as dizygotic (DZ) or fraternal twins. Genetically, DZ twins do not differ from singleton brother–brother, sister–sister or brother–sister pairs, that is they share on average 50% of their genetic material. Opposite-sex (OS) twins are always DZ twins.

By comparing the resemblance in traits between MZ and DZ twins, we can decompose familial resemblance into unique environmental (E), shared environmental (C), additive (A) genetic and dominant (D) genetic factors [9]. If the resemblance in a trait within MZ pairs is larger than in DZ pairs, this suggests that additive and possibly dominant genetic factors influence the trait. If the resemblance in the trait is as large in DZ twins as it is in MZ twins, this points to shared environmental factors as the cause of family resemblance. The extent to which MZ twins do not resemble each other is ascribed to the unique (or non-shared) environmental factors. These include all unique experiences such as differential jobs or lifestyle, accidents or other life events, and in childhood differential treatment by the parents and non-shared peers.

In the classical twin design, we can only estimate three components of variance at the same time (A, C and E, or A, D and E). Therefore, one needs to make the assumption that either C or D is absent. The absence of dominance can be reasonably assumed if the DZ correlations are not much lower than half the MZ correlation. In the absence of shared environmental effects, the DZ correlations should not be much higher than half the MZ correlations. It is also possible to fully estimate both common environmental and dominance effects by adding parents and offspring of twins to the classical twin design [10].

Twin researchers typically use structural equation modelling (SEM) to estimate the relative contribution of A, D, C and E to the individual differences in the trait. In SEM, the relationships between several latent unobserved variables (e.g. genetic and environmental factors) and observed variables are summarised by a series of equations. Additional equations can specify the correlation between the latent genetic and environmental factors if these are known. It is possible to derive the variance–covariance matrix implied by the total set of equations ('the model') using covariance algebra. When the complexity and number of the equations increases, the structural equation model can be formulated more easily by application of path-tracing rules on the complete representation of all relationships between observed and unobserved variables in a so-called path diagram. An example of a model with A, C and E is depicted in Figure 3.1, where depressive symptoms had been measured with the Beck Depression Inventory in DZ and MZ twin pairs [11].

Using maximum likelihood estimation, we can now iteratively test the fit of the expected covariances/variances implied by Figure 3.1 to the actual observed covariances/variances in a sample of hundreds or thousands of twins over a range of possible values for the path coefficients. From the best-fitting model we take the estimates for the path coefficients (e.g. a, c and e) and determine the relative contribution of the latent A, C, E factors to the total variance in depressive symptoms. Heritability of these symptoms, defined as the relative proportion of the total variance explained by genetic factors, is obtained as the ratio of $a^2/(a^2 + e^2 + c^2)$. The heritability coefficient

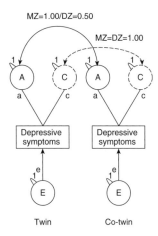

Figure 3.1 Variance decomposition in twin studies using a path model. DZ – dizygotic; MZ – monozygotic. The correlation between the latent genetic factors are set to unity for MZ twins and to 0.5 for DZ twins. For both twins, shared environmental factors are correlated with unity. Variances of the latent factors are standardised to be unity. Path coefficients a, c, e can be estimated by a maximum likelihood estimation procedure that optimally fits the expected variance and covariances to the observed variance in depressive symptoms and the observed cross-twin covariances in MZ and DZ twin pairs.

(abbreviated as h^2) can also be expressed as a percentage by multiplying this ratio by 100. For depressive symptoms in adult Dutch twins, measured repeatedly over time, this heritability varied between 42% and 53% for females and between 39% and 46% for males [11].

It is important to stress that the parameter estimates derived from twin studies are to be understood as applying to a population, not an individual. Just like the mean or the standard deviation of depressive symptoms, the heritability coefficient is a descriptive statistic for the sampled population, and should be regarded as such. It may or may not generalise to other samples. A second note of caution is that the twin method assumes that twins in the same household are exposed to shared environmental factors to the same extent whether they are MZ or DZ ('equal environment assumption'). If this is not the case, and MZ twin pairs are exposed to more similar environments than DZ pairs, then any excess similarity in MZ pairs compared with DZ pairs may be the result of shared environmental rather than genetic factors. The equal environment assumption has been a main target for sceptics of the twin method. All of its empirical tests, however, have shown that the assumption holds very well even for behavioural traits (e.g. intelligence, personality) that should be most sensitive to its violation [12–15].

Heritability of MDD and Depressive Symptoms

A meta-analysis of twin (and family) studies estimated the heritability of adult MDD around 40% [16] and this estimate is strikingly stable across different countries [17, 18]. If measurement error due to unreliability is taken into account by analysing MDD assessed on two occasions, heritability estimates increase to 66% [19]. Twin studies in children further show that there is already a large genetic contribution to depressive symptoms in youth, with heritability estimates varying between 50% and 80% [20–22]. Genetic factors influencing symptoms of anxiety and depression appear to be partly stable from childhood till at least 20 years of age, although new genetic factors may come online in early adulthood [23, 24]. Depressive symptoms in adults, measured by various instruments, show a heritability of around 40% and this estimate varies little across countries [11, 25, 26]. Stability in these adult depressive symptoms is almost entirely attributable to the same set of genetic factors [27–29].

Heritability of CAD and CAD Risk Factors

Cardiovascular research in twin samples has suggested a clear-cut genetic contribution to hypertension ($h^2 = 61\%$) [30], fatal stroke ($h^2 = 32\%$) [31] and CAD ($h^2 = 57\%$ in males and 38% in females) [32].

The genetic contribution to these disease end points results from the joint effects of risk genes on the many biological and behavioural risk factors that impact on the atherosclerotic process. Genetic factors have been shown to contribute substantially to smoking [33, 34], physical inactivity [35, 36], body mass index [37], type 2 diabetes [38], systolic and diastolic blood pressure [30, 39] and plasma low density lipoprotein (LDL)-C and high-density lipoprotein (HDL)-C levels [40]. Heritability estimates for these established risk factors are 50% or higher in most adult twin samples and these estimates remain remarkably similar across the adult life span [41–43]. Population variance in a number of other suspected risk factors, including glucose intolerance [44–46], insulin resistance [47], C-reactive protein (CRP) [48], pro-inflammatory cytokines [49,50], haemostasis [51,52], resting cardiac autonomic control [53–55] and autonomic reactivity to stress [56], also shows significant genetic contribution, with heritability estimates of at least 30%.

Bivariate Heritability

The crucial question is whether the genetic factors underlying MDD also play a role in CAD and CAD risk factors. To test for an overlap in the genetic factors, a bivariate extension of the structural equation model for twin data can be used [57]. This allows a whole new set of hypotheses to be tested, because the observed information now includes all possible cross-twin cross-trait correlations, for instance the correlation of depressive symptoms in a twin measured by the Beck Depression Inventory with the interleukin (IL)-6 levels in his/her co-twin [26]. If the depressive symptoms in a twin predict the IL-6 level in his/her co-twin, this can only be explained by an underlying factor that affects both depression and IL-6 levels and is shared by members of a family. If the prediction is much stronger in MZ than in DZ twins, this signals that the underlying factor is their shared genetic make-up, rather than their shared (family) environment.

Figure 3.2 illustrates an extended path model that can be used to compute bivariate heritability. Common genetic factor A influences the depressive symptoms, including the possible pleiotropic genes that influence inflammation. The specific genetic factor As contains the genetic factors that are specific to inflammation only. Path coefficient a_{11} quantifies the effect of genetic factor A on the depressive symptoms; a_{21} quantifies the potential pleiotropic genetic effect of A on IL-6. Coefficient a_{22} quantifies the effect of specific genetic factor As

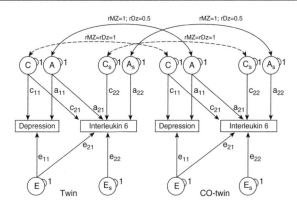

Figure 3.2 Bivariate twin model to test the sharing of genetic and environmental factors between two traits. DZ – dizygotic; MZ – monozygotic.

on IL-6. If a_{21} is zero and a_{22} is significantly different from zero, the association between depression and inflammation does not derive from the same genetic factor and there is no evidence for pleiotropy. In a similar way, path coefficients $e_{11}, c_{11}, e_{21}, c_{21}, e_{22}$ and c_{22} quantify the effects of common and specific factors E and C on the two traits. If c_{21} is non-significant, but c_{22} significantly different from zero, the association between depressive symptoms and inflammation does not derive from the same common environmental factor.

Alternatively, the bivariate twin model in Figure 3.2 can be used to decompose a phenotypic correlation between two traits into its three possible sources: overlapping genetic, overlapping shared environmental or overlapping unique environmental factors. The word 'overlapping' can be defined more precisely as the correlation between the latent genetic (R_A), shared environmental (R_C) or unique environmental (R_E) factors influencing depressive symptoms (A, C, E) and IL-6 (As, Cs, Es). Using the heritability of the two traits together with their genetic correlation, it is possible to compute the contribution of genetic factors to the observed association between the two traits.

It is important to note clearly here that genetic correlations do not prove the existence of pleiotropy, because genes that influence MDD may, through causal effects of MDD on CAD risk, also become 'CAD genes'. The absence of a genetic correlation, however, can be used to falsify the existence of genetic pleiotropy. For instance, the hypothesis that genetic pleiotropy explains part of the association between depressive symptoms and IL-6 requires the genetic correlation between these traits to be significantly different from zero. Furthermore, since we assume that the pleiotropic factors increase the risk for depression and create a pro-inflammatory state, the genetic correlation should have a positive value. A negative genetic correlation would signal that genes that increase the risk for depression decrease the risk for higher IL-6 levels, which would go against the genetic pleiotropy hypothesis.

Figure 3.2 was modelled after the study of Su et al. [26], who tested pleiotropy as a possible source of the association of depressive symptoms with Il-6 in 188 twin pairs of the Vietnam Era Twin (VET) Registry. The genetic correlation between depressive symptoms and IL-6 was found to be positive and significant ($R_A = 0.22$, $p = 0.046$) and increased to 0.27 after correction for the Framingham risk score, obesity and physical inactivity. Genetic factors explained 93% of the covariation between depressive symptoms and IL-6. This is compatible with the idea that genetic pleiotropy is causing part of the association between these two traits.

MDD and CAD

Genetic correlations can also be computed on dichotomous traits, such as MDD or CAD diagnoses, by using tetrachoric correlations that map the affected/unaffected status into an underlying liability [57]. In 1561 male MZ pairs and 1170 male DZ pairs from the same VET Registry, a genetic correlation of $+0.19$ was found between depressive symptoms and hypertension and a genetic correlation of $+0.42$ between depressive symptoms and self-reported heart disease [58]. Trivariate modelling showed that additive genetic factors common to all three disorders explained the total heritability (64%) of heart disease, 7% of the variance in risk for hypertension (total $h^2 = 57\%$) and 8% of the variance in risk for depression symptoms (total $h^2 = 37\%$). Importantly, the environmental correlations between depression and heart disease, and between depression and hypertension, were *not* significant.

Why is this important? Because the pattern of genetic and environmental correlations can be used to falsify the causal hypothesis. A strong prediction from the main causal hypothesis in the MDD–CAD morbidity is that *all* factors that influence MDD should also influence CAD. Hence, both genetic and environmental factors that increase MDD must, through the causal chain, also increase the risk for CAD. Translating this to the structural equation models used on twin data, this means that causal hypotheses predict that both the genetic (R_A) and environmental $(R_C$ and/or $R_E)$ correlations between MD and CAD must be significantly different from zero. The pattern found by Scherrer et al. [58] falsifies the causal hypothesis $(R_E = 0)$, whereas it does not falsify the pleiotropic hypothesis $(R_A > 0)$.

Using a much larger sample of 15 285 Swedish twin pairs participating in the Screening Across the Lifespan Twin (SALT) study, Kendler et al. [59] also reported a significant genetic correlation between MDD and CAD, but important differences were found between males and females. These were further qualified by the age of onset of CAD. The genetic correlation between MDD and CAD in men was positive in the younger twins $(R_A = +0.12)$ with mean birth year 1953 but *negative* in older twins in the sample with mean birth year 1930 $(R_A = -0.16)$. In women, the genetic correlation between MDD and CAD was $+0.16$ across all age groups. In the male twins, a significant environmental correlation was found $(R_E = 0.13)$, whereas in younger male twins and in women of all ages the environmental correlations were close to zero $(R_E = +0.04)$.

These results suggest that early-onset CAD in males and both early- and late-onset CAD in females were associated with MDD largely through shared genetic factors. This finding is compatible with the genetic pleiotropy hypothesis. In the older male twins, however, environmental factors were the main source of comorbidity. This may reflect another important finding in this study, namely that short-acting factors appeared more important in explaining the comorbidity for males than for females. Perhaps in late-onset male CAD, short-acting environmental factors are essential for MDD–CAD comorbidity. Genetic pleiotropy could be limited to women or early-onset CAD in men. However, the very low prevalence of MDD cases in the older twins in this sample suggests that further confirmation is needed of this finding before it is quoted as a solid falsification of genetic pleiotropy.

MDD and CAD Risk Factors

Because the broad categories of CAD outcomes, such as angina, myocardial infarction (MI), or sudden cardiac death (SCD), reflect a heterogeneous set of disease aetiologies, multivariate twin studies of MDD or depressive symptom counts have also been performed with many intermediate CAD risk factors, both behavioural and physiological. Vaccarino et al. [60] tested the integrity of the coronary microcirculation using positron emission tomography (PET)-based measures of coronary flow reserve (CFR) in twins from the VET study. They used a slightly different strategy to test for genetic pleiotropy, known as the discordant twin design. MZ and DZ twins were selected to be discordant for lifetime MDD, such that one twin was affected at the time of CFR scanning whereas the other twin was not. In the entire sample a significant association was found between CFR and MDD. When contrasting the affected and unaffected members of MDD discordant twin pairs, only the affected member of the DZ twin pairs had a lower CFR than the unaffected member. MZ twins, even if discordant for depression, did *not* show different CFR. Since MZ twins are 100% matched on their segregating genes, the within-pair difference in MDD arises through environmental factors. These factors apparently influence only MDD, but do not influence CFR, which refutes a causal effect of MDD on CFR. DZ twins are only 50% matched and the discordance in MDD may reflect risk genes in one twin that were not segregated to the other twin. These risk genes apparently also have a detrimental influence on the coronary microcirculation.

Twin and family studies have further addressed genetic pleiotropy in the association of depression with metabolic abnormalities such as abdominal obesity, insulin resistance, hyperglycaemia and dyslipidaemia. These characteristics, often with the addition of hypertension, are usually clustered as the 'metabolic syndrome' (MetS). MetS affects approximately one-fifth of the adult population and has repeatedly been shown to be associated with depressive symptomatology [61, 62]. In 150 male twins from the VET Registry, a MetS factor score was composed from the mean arterial blood pressure, body mass index, waist–hip ratio, triglyceride levels and fasting glucose. Participants also completed the Center for Epidemiology

Studies Depression Scale (CES-D), a 20-item scale assessing depressive symptoms. Genetic effects did not contribute significantly to the association between depressive symptoms and the MetS factor score. Instead the correlation between depressive symptoms and the metabolic factor ($r = 0.16$) was mainly caused by unique environmental factors. This clearly argues against pleiotropy, at least with regard to MetS. At the same time it argues against causal effects of depression, because under the causal hypothesis the genetic factors underlying the heritability of depression should also have affected the MetS. Some caution is required in interpreting this study, in view of the modest sample size. When the correlation is low at the trait level (0.16), many hundreds of twins may be required to detect significant R_A, R_C and R_E [63].

Using a family-based approach, which employs the same underlying biometrical principles as the twin study, López-León et al. [64] tested the source of the co-occurrence of symptoms of depression and cardiovascular risk factors in a much larger sample of 2383 individuals from a genetically isolated population in the Netherlands. Symptoms of depression were assessed using the CES-D. Assessment of metabolic risk factors included systolic and diastolic blood pressure, fasting glucose levels, HDL, LDL and total cholesterol (CHOL) levels as well as the CHOL/HDL ratio. Significant genetic correlations were found between CES-D scores and total plasma cholesterol ($R_A = 0.30$), LDL ($R_A = 0.31$) and total cholesterol/HDL ratios ($R_A = 0.25$). Environmental correlations were either close to zero or in the opposite direction (R_E CHOL $= -0.16$; R_E LDL $= -0.15$). These findings argue in favour of genetic pleiotropy as the explanation for the association between MDD and an unfavourable lipid spectrum.

Additional evidence for pleiotropy comes from the area of inflammation. Using the same discordant design as described for CFR above, Vaccarino et al. [65] showed that the white blood cell count (WBC) and levels of myeloperoxidase (MPO), an enzyme produced by activated leucocytes as part of the innate immune response, were higher in twins who had an MDD diagnosis than twins without such a diagnosis, even after correcting for body mass index, physical activity, history of heart disease and the Framingham risk score. Separate testing of MZ and DZ within pair contrasts showed that this was exclusively based on the DZ twins, not on the MZ twins, arguing in favour of genetic pleiotropy. In this same sample, adjusted levels of fibrinogen, CRP, tumour necrosis factor (TNF)-α, the TNF-α soluble receptor 2 (TNFRII) and IL-6 were not significantly different between affected and unaffected DZ twins. However, this may in part reflect the loss of power that is incurred by selecting only the discordant twin pairs, rather than computing a genetic correlation across the full twin sample. For instance, in a reanalysis of the same VET sample, Su et al. [26] showed that IL-6 *did* have a significant genetic correlation to MDD, whereas the environmental correlation was non-significant.

A very important, and perhaps underestimated, source of pleiotropy in the association of MDD and CAD are the major behavioural risk factors for CAD: smoking and physical inactivity. These factors are sometimes considered 'environmental', but twin studies have shown that such behaviours have a strong genetic component [33–35].

For smoking, various studies have shown that it shares part of this genetic component with MDD. In 8169 male twins from the VET Registry, genetic factors influencing MDD also strongly influenced nicotine dependence [66]. However, among the 237 MZ pairs discordant for MDD, it was additionally shown that the depressed probands were more likely to have a lifetime history of nicotine dependence than their non-depressed co-twins. These findings are compatible with a causal effect of MDD on nicotine dependence (or vice versa) as well as with genetic pleiotropy in adult men. Additional support for a genetic correlation in the presence of support for causal effects of MDD comes from 287 MZ and 441 DZ twins participating in the National Longitudinal Study of Adolescent Health [67]. In this adolescent sample, a significant genetic correlation was found in females (0.62) but not in males, whereas environmental factors for depressive symptoms and smoking were correlated in both males and females (0.23). Finally, a large sample of Finnish twins reported a significant genetic correlation between smoking behaviour in 1975 or 1981 and depressive symptoms in 1990 ($R_A = 0.25$), but only in males [68].

For the association between MDD and physical inactivity, the dominant hypothesis has not been that MDD causes a reduction in regular exercise, but instead that regular exercise may act as a protective factor against mood disorders. This popular idea of exercise as a buffer against stress and a boost for psychological well-being was supported by various studies addressing the association in longitudinal designs, showing that regular leisure time exercise at baseline was associated with less depression and anxiety at follow-up [69–77]. As outlined before, this does not rule out genetic pleiotropy, and we used the twin method to perform a rigorous test of this popular hypothesis [78]. The crucial prediction from the causal hypothesis – that there are both genetic and environmental correlations between exercise and anxious/depressive symptoms – was tested in 8558 twins and their family members using their longitudinal data across 2-, 4-, 7-, 9- and 11-year follow-up periods.

In spite of sufficient statistical power, we found only the genetic correlation to be significant (ranging between -0.16 and -0.44 for different symptom scales and different time-lags). The environmental correlations were essentially zero. This means that the environmental factors that cause a person to take up exercise do not cause lower anxiety or depressive symptoms in that person, currently or at any future time point. In contrast, the genetic factors that cause a person to take up exercise also cause lower anxiety or depressive symptoms in that person, at the present and all future time points. This pattern of results falsifies the causal hypothesis and leaves genetic pleiotropy as the most likely source for the association between exercise and lower levels of anxiety and depressive symptoms in the population at large.

Table 3.1 summarises the genetic and environmental correlations from the studies reviewed above. Taken together, these studies support the idea that genetic pleiotropy may be a factor contributing to the increased risk for CAD in subjects suffering from MDD or reporting high counts of depressive symptoms. The absence of environmental correlations in the presence of significant genetic correlations for a number of the CAD risk factors (CFR, cholesterol, inflammation and regular exercise) suggests that pleiotropy is the sole reason for the association between MDD and these CAD risk factors, whereas for other CAD risk factors (e.g. smoking) and CAD incidence itself, pleiotropy may coexist with causal effects. There are likely to be important further nuances, related to age and birth cohort effects, and male and female differences. Ethnicity may be a further modifier and it should be noted that the available twin studies consisted largely of individuals with a Caucasian background.

Table 3.1 Bivariate heritability for depression and CAD risk

Sample	Depression variable	CAD variable	Genetic correlation (R_A)	Environmental correlations (R_E/R_C)	Reference
1561 male MZ pairs and 1170 DZ pairs from the VET Registry > 90% Caucasian, age 41.9 ± 2.7	Telephone administration DIS-3R for lifetime depression (DSM-III-R)	Self-reported heart disease (angina, MI, CAD, heart surgery), N = 124 cases Self-reported hypertension, N = 1264 cases	R_A = **0.42** R_A = **0.19**	R_E = 0 R_E = 0	[58]
15 285 male and female twin pairs (26.4% MZ) from the Swedish Twin Registry Caucasian, age 57.3 ± 11.5	Telephone administration CIDI-SF for lifetime depression (DSM-IV)	ICD coded diagnoses from Cause of Death Register (MI, angina, CAD, IHD, heart surgery), N = 3099 cases	Young men: R_A = **0.12** Young women: R_A = **0.16** Older men: R_A = **−0.16** Older women: R_A = **0.16**	R_E = **0.13** R_E = 0.04 R_E = **0.13** R_E = 0.04	[59]

(Continued)

Table 3.1 (Continued)

Sample	Depression variable	CAD variable	Genetic correlation (R_A)	Environmental correlations (R_E/R_C)	Reference
135 male MZ and 101 male DZ twins from the VET Registry > 90% Caucasian Age 54.3 ± 2.8 53 MDD discordant pairs 183 MDD free pairs	Structured clinical interview for lifetime depression (DSM-IV)	CFR (PET-derived myocardial blood flow after adenosine infusion minus blood flow at rest)	Affected twin in MDD discordant DZ pairs: CFR 15% lower $R_A > \mathbf{0}$	Affected twin in MDD discordant MZ pairs: no CFR difference $R_E = 0$	[60]
76 male MZ and 73 male DZ twin pairs from the VET Registry > 90% Caucasian Age 63.1 ± 2.9	CES-D (survey), current depressive symptoms	Metabolic factor based on blood pressure, BMI, waist–hip ratio, triglycerides, and glucose	$R_A = 0.0$	$R_E = \mathbf{0.48}$	[121]

2383 offspring from 28 founder families in a genetically isolated population in the Netherlands Caucasian Age 48.7 ± 15.1	CES-D (survey), current depressive symptoms	Blood pressure Glucose CHOL LDL CHOL/HDL ratio	R_A = −0.15 R_A = 0.12 R_A = **0.30** R_A = **0.31** R_A = **0.25**	R_E = −0.03 R_E = 0.05 R_E = **−0.16** R_E = **−0.15** R_E = 0.06	[80]
93 male MZ pairs and 87 male DZ pairs from the VET Registry > 90% Caucasian Age 54.3 ± 2.8 67 (32 DZ) were MDD discordant pairs	Structured clinical interview for lifetime depression (DSM-IV)	TNF-α, TNFRII, CRP fibrinogen, IL-6, MPO WBC	Affected twin in MDD discordant DZ pairs: MPO 77% higher WBC 18% higher R_A > **0**	Affected twin in MDD discordant MZ pairs: no significant MPO and WBC differences R_E = 0	[65]
108 male MZ and 80 male DZ twins from the VET Registry > 90% Caucasian Age 54.9 ± 2.7	Structured clinical interview for lifetime depression (DSM-IV)	IL-6 CRP	R_A = **0.27** R_A = 0	R_E = 0.02 R_E = 0	[26]

(Continued)

Table 3.1 (Continued)

Sample	Depression variable	CAD variable	Genetic correlation (R_A)	Environmental correlations (R_E/R_C)	Reference
8169 male twins of the VET Registry > 90% Caucasian Age 44.6 ± 2.8	Telephone administration DIS-3R for lifetime depression (DSM-IIIR)	Interview based daily smoking nicotine dependence	$R_A = $ **0.17** $R_A = $ **0.70**	$R_E = $ n.a. $R_E = $ n.a. Affected twin in MDD discordant MZ pairs: more nicotine dependence $R_E > $ **0**	[66]
287 MZ and 441 DZ twins from the National Longitudinal Study of Adolescent Health Mixed ethnicity Age 16.1 ± 1.6	CES-D (in-home interview), current depressive symptoms	Current smoking behaviour	Female: $R_A = $ **0.62** Male: $R_A = 0$	Female: $R_E = $ **0.23** Male: $R_E = $ **0.23**	[67]

10 977 twins from the Finnish Twin Cohort Age 35.2 Caucasian 172 MZ pairs, 407 DZ smoking discordant pairs	Beck Depression Inventory, 21 item version (survey)	Smoking behaviour from longitudinal surveys	Female: R_A = 0 Male: R_A = **0.25**	Female: R_E = n.a. Male: R_E = 0.10 Smoking twin in smoke discordant MZ pairs (M + F): more depressive symptoms R_E > **0**	[68]
1195 MZ and 1352 DZ twin pairs from the Netherland Twin Registry Age 27.9 ± 8.0 Caucasian	Young Adult Self Report Scale, anxious-depression subscale (survey)	Regular leisure time exercise	Female: R_A = **−0.22** Male: R_A = **−0.24**	Female: R_E =0.02 Male: R_E = − 0.03	[122]

n.a. – estimates not given in the paper.

Bold – correlations significant at p <0.05.

MZ – monozygotic; DZ – dizygotic; DIS-3R – Diagnostic Interview Schedule Version 3; MI – myocardial infarction; CAD – coronary artery disease; CIDI-SF – Composite International Diagnostic Interview Short Form; MDD – major depressive disorder; CFR – coronary flow reserve; CES-D – Center for Epidemiology Studies Depression Scale; BMI – body mass index; CHOL – cholesterol; CRP – C-reactive protein; MPO – myeloperoxidase; WBC – white blood cell count.

GENETIC ASSOCIATION STUDIES

Although twin studies show that MDD and CAD potentially share genetic risk factors, these factors are modelled as latent factors, and the actual gene networks that harbour the allelic variants underlying both diseases are left unspecified. Identification of these genes could help elucidate the pathophysiology of both classes of disease, and also provide a more direct biological account of the hypothesised genetic pleiotropy.

Until recently, the main gene-finding strategy was through the use of candidate genes. Candidate gene association studies simply test whether a particular allele in a candidate gene and a trait co-occur above chance level, given the frequency of the allele and the distribution of the trait in the population [66]. The *a priori* selection of genes may be based on the biological role of the gene in a causative pathway (physiological candidate) and/or its location close to a peak from a linkage study (positional candidate). The variants to be typed within the gene – for example single nucleotide polymorphisms (SNPs), repeat polymorphisms or insertion/deletion polymorphisms – are prioritised by their location within coding, promoter or splice regions, or, if known, their functional effects on the gene product or on gene expression.

Although previous studies have suggested that association can be detected even in modestly sized samples, standard power calculations show that up to 1000 participants are required to detect gene main effects with small to medium-effect sizes [79]. This requires a large investment in sample collection and this effort must be weighed against an important disadvantage of the candidate gene approach: that it entirely capitalises on existing biological disease models. Many of the hundreds or thousands of genes relevant to the disease may not have been properly functionally annotated or reside in pathways that have not been linked to the disease before.

Increasingly, gene-finding attempts in large samples have used the more agnostic strategy of a genome-wide association (GWA) study. GWA studies exploit the development of affordable, high-accuracy, high-throughput genotyping technologies for the Human Genome Sequencing Project. Between 100 000 and 1 million SNPs scattered across the entire genome are genotyped for each individual in a study.

Together with the increased information on the haplotype structure of the world's main populations obtained from the HapMap project, these SNP data can be used to test genetic association to disease or disease risk factors on a genome-wide scale, without any *a priori* assumptions on the biological pathways involved.

Genes Associated with Depression

Almost all gene-finding studies on MDD have used a candidate gene approach. Table 3.2 presents a list of genes that have been found to be significantly associated at least once to clinical depression, depressive symptom scores, compiled from recent reviews [80–82]. Such lists are by their nature illustrative rather than definitive, because ongoing progress in the understanding of the biology of depression will keep generating new candidates.

Table 3.2 Genes used in candidate gene studies on MDD or depressive symptoms

AACT	14q32.1
ACE	17q23.3
ACSL4	Xq22.3-q23
ADCY9	16p13.3
ADORA2A	22q11.23
ADRA2A	10q24-q26
ADRB1	10q24-q26
AGTR1	3q21-q25
APOE	19q13.2
AR	Xq11.2-q12
AVPR1B	1q32
BCR	22q11.23
BDNF	11p13
C5orf20 (DCNP1)	5q31.1
CAMKK2	12q24.2
CCK	3p22-p21.3
CCKAR	4p15.1-p15.2
CCKBR	11p15.4
CCL2	17q11.2-q12
CGF1	Xp11.22-qter

(Continued)

Table 3.2 (*Continued*)

CHRM2	7q31-q35
CHRNA7	15q13.1
CLOCK	4q12
CNR1	6q14-q15
CNTF	11q12.2
COMT	22q11.21
CRHBP	5q11.2-q13.3
CRHR1	17q12-q22
CRHR2	7p14.3
CTLA4	2q33
CYP2C9	10q24
CYP2D6	22q13.1
DAOA	13q34
DDC	7p12.2
DISC1	1q42.1
DRD1	5q35.1
DRD2	11q23
DRD3	3q13.3
DRD4	11p15.5
DRD5	4p16.1
DTNBP1	6p22.3
DUSP6	12q22-q23
ESR1	6q25.1
ESR2	14q23.2
FKBP5	6p21.3-p21.2
FZD3	8p21
GABRA1	5q34-q35
GABRA3	Xq28
GABRA5	15q11.2-q12
GABRA6	5q34
GAD1	2q31
GMIP	19p12-p11
GNAL	18p11.22-p11.21
GNAS	20q13.3
GNB3	12p13
GPBAR1	2q35
GPR50	Xq28
GYPA	4q28.2-q31.1
HP	16q22.1
HTR1A	5q11.2-q13
HTR1B	6q13
HTR2A	13q14-q21

Table 3.2 (*Continued*)

HTR2C	Xq24
HTR3A	11q23.1
HTR3B	11q23.1
HTR5A	7q36.1
HTR6	1p36-p35
IL10	1q31-q32
IL1B	2q14
IL6	7p21
LBP	20q11.23-q12
LHPP	10q26.13
LRP	12q13-q14
M6PR	12p13
MAOA	Xp11.3
MAOB	Xp11.23
MTHFR	1p36.3
NGFR	17q21-q22
NOS1	12q24.2-q24.31
NOS3	7q36
NPY	7p15.1
NR3C1	5q31.3
NR3C2	4q31.1
OASL	12q24.2
OPRD1	1p36.1-p34.3
OPRK1	8q11.2
OPRM1	6q24-q25
P2RX4	12q24.32
P2RX7	12q24
PAM	5q14-q21
PDE10A	6q26
PDE11A	2q31.2
PDE2A	11q13.4
PDE5A	4q25-q27
PDE6C	10q24
PDE9A	21q22.3
PENK	8q23-q24
PLA2G2A	1p35
PLA2G4A	1q25
POMC	2p23.3
SLC6A2	16q12.2
SLC6A4	17q11.1-q12

(*Continued*)

Table 3.2 (*Continued*)

TAC1	7q21-q22
TACR1	2p12
TFCP2	12q13
TH	11p15.5
TNF	6p21.3
TPH1	11p15.3-p14
TPH2	12q21.1
WFS1	4p16

By far the most tested polymorphism in psychiatric genetics is a 43-base pair insertion or deletion in the promoter region of the serotonin transporter gene (5HTT, renamed SLC6A4). About 55% of Caucasians carry a long allele (L) with 16 repeat units. The short allele (S, with 14 repeat units) of this length polymorphism repeat (LPR) reduces transcriptional efficiency, resulting in decreased serotonin transporter expression and function [83]. Because serotonin plays a key role in one of the major theories of MDD [84], and because the most prescribed antidepressants act directly on this transporter, 5HTT is an obvious candidate gene for this disorder.

The dearth of studies attempting to associate the 5HTTLPR to MDD or related personality traits tells a revealing story about the fate of most candidate genes in psychiatric genetics. Many conflicting findings have been reported, and the two largest studies failed to link the 5HTTLPR to depressive symptoms or clinical MDD [85, 86]. Even at the level of reviews and meta-analyses, conflicting conclusions have been drawn about the role of this polymorphism in the development of MDD [87, 88]. The initially promising explanation for discrepant findings – potential interactive effects of the 5HTTLPR and stressful life events [89] – did not survive meta-analysis [90]. Some of the unrest may have to be attributed to the difficulty of correctly genotyping this repeat polymorphism. In spite of 5HTTLPR's popularity, the genotyping assay presents a non-trivial challenge for most laboratories and there is considerable bias toward S allele identification [91]. In addition, only the more recent studies have accounted for the presence of the G allele at an A/G SNP rs25531 that lies within the L allele, which makes the L (denoted L_G) functionally equivalent to the S allele [92]. Even after all the work carried out, we cannot trust this gene as an 'MDD gene'. At the same time, new variants are still being uncovered in the 5HTT gene [91], so its importance for MDD can still not be ruled out.

Across the board, overlooking the wealth of candidate gene studies on MDD, one is inclined to conclude that this approach has failed to unambiguously identify genetic variants involved in MDD [86, 90, 93, 94]. Hope is now focused on the newer GWA approach. At the time of writing, only two GWA studies had been published on MDD [81, 95]. A study on 1359 recurrent MDD patients and 1782 control subjects [95] reinforced the gene coding for an mGluR7 (GRM7) as a plausible gene for MDD, in keeping with the emergence of glutamate signalling as a potential target for the treatment of mood disorders [96]. A study on 1738 MDD cases and 1802 control subjects selected to be at low liability for MDD [81, 97] presented evidence for an effect of variation in a gene on chromosome 7 coding for the presynaptic protein piccolo (PCLO). PCLO's association to MDD has since been independently replicated [98].

Of note is that both GWA studies did not reach the required p-value threshold of 10^{-8} that is considered to be a genuine association. GWA studies use this stern significance level to deal with the multiple testing problem inherent in testing for about 1 million independent genomic regions. Consequently, the studies that involve 'only' a few thousands of individuals may still have been underpowered to discover common genetic variants with modest to low effect sizes (e.g. genotypic odds ratios between 1.05 and 1.30). One way forward is to collate samples of many tens of thousands of MDD patients and controls through large-scale pooling of data across many different centres and studies. Such collaborative attempts are currently under way for MDD [99].

In the meantime, we have explored an alternative strategy to increase the chances to detect relevant gene networks in MDD from the first GWA data. In this so-called pathway analysis approach, we applied far more lenient thresholds for significance but in exchange demanded that the data 'make sense' in the existing corpus of knowledge in molecular biology. To do so, we combined our GWA results on MDD [81] with the rapidly expanding information on patterns of co-expression of genes, protein–protein interactions, and shared biological functions of gene products and co-citation of genes and (disease) phenotypes as, for example, defined within Ingenuity Knowledge Base. Our pathway analysis suggested that the set of genes associated with MDD at a p-value of 0.05 was significantly enriched for inflammatory genes, in particular the TNF gene and genes coding for molecules interacting with TNF-α. This finding supports the cytokine hypothesis of depression, which postulates a low-grade chronic pro-inflammatory response to be a driving force behind the illness [7, 100].

Genes Associated with CAD and CAD Risk Factors

Table 3.3 presents a list of GWA-derived genes for CAD outcomes (MI, SCD, stroke) and CAD risk factors (diabetes, obesity, blood pressure, lipids, smoking, exercise) compiled from a regularly updated Web-based catalogue of published GWA studies (www. genome.gov/gwastudies) combined with recent reviews and GWA studies [101–110]. Clearly, there have been far more GWA studies carried out in this field than for MDD, and with greater success. For instance, over 35 loci have been detected to influence LDL, HDL, CHOL or triglyceride levels [109]. The GWA approach has also been successfully applied to type 2 diabetes [103, 111, 112] and continuously distributed traits such as fasting insulin and glucose [106] and obesity [104, 113]. The heritability of blood pressure has proven to be a hard nut to crack, but with the ongoing increase in the scale of international collaboration, and parallel increases in sample sizes to over 70 000 subjects, GWA studies are starting to pay off here too [101, 114]. Finally, GWA studies on major behavioural risk factors such as smoking and regular exercise have yielded a first glimpse of the genes that influence these behaviours [115–118].

Many of the genes detected were not on any *a priori* candidate gene list, confirming the power of GWA to identify new biology. For instance, only four of the 24 type 2 diabetes-associated variants have been identified through candidate gene studies. At the same time, a number of candidate genes for lipid metabolism held up very well in

Table 3.3 Genes with significant SNPs in genome-wide association for CAD and CAD risk factors

Atrial fibrillation	PITX2
BMI	BDNF
BMI	FTO
BMI	GNPDA2
BMI	INSIG2
BMI	KCTD15
BMI	MC4R
BMI	MTCH2
BMI	NEGR1
BMI	PCSK1
BMI	SH2B1
BMI	TMEM18
BMI, extreme	PCSK1
Coronary artery calcification	CDKN2A, CDKN2B
Coronary artery calcification	PHACTR1
CAD; MI	LC22A3, LPAL2, LPA
CAD; MI	MRAS
DBP	ATP2B1
DBP	c10orf107
DBP	CACNB2
DBP	CSK, ULK3
DBP	CYP1A2
DBP	FGF5
DBP	SH2B3
DBP	TBX3-TBX5
DBP	ULK4
DBP	ZNF652
HDL	ABCA1
HDL	ANGPTL4
HDL	APOA1-C3-A4–A5
HDL	CETP
HDL	CTCF, PRMT8
HDL	FADS1-3 cluster
HDL	GALNT2
HDL	HNF4A
HDL	LCAT
HDL	LIPC
HDL	LIPG
HDL	LPL
HDL	MADD, FOLH1

(*Continued*)

Table 3.3 (*Continued*)

HDL	MMAB,MVK
HDL	PLTP
HDL	TTC39B
HDL, triglycerides	APOB
HDL, triglycerides	LPL
HOMA IR; insulin	IGF1
HOMA-B; glucose	ADRA2A
HOMA-B; glucose	CRY2
HOMA-B; glucose	FADS1-3 cluster
HOMA-B; glucose	FAM148B (NLF2)
HOMA-B; glucose	G6PC2
HOMA-B; glucose	GLIS3
HOMA-B; glucose	MADD, FOLH1
HOMA-B; glucose	SLC2A2
Hypertension	ATP2B1
Intracranial aneurysm	BOLL, PLCL1
Intracranial aneurysm	CDKN2A, CDKN2B
Intracranial aneurysm	SOX17
LDL	ABCG8
LDL	APOB
LDL	APOE-APOC1/C4/C2
LDL	CELSR2/PSRC1/SORT1
LDL	DNAH11
LDL	HMGCR
LDL	HNF1A
LDL	LDLR
LDL	MAFB
LDL	NCAN, CILP2, PBX4
LDL	PCSK9
LDL	TIMD4, HAVCR1
LV internal diastolic dimensions	C6orf204,PLN
LV internal diastolic dimensions	SLC35F1
LV mass	CALM2
LV mass	NOVA1
LV systolic dysfunction	HN1L
LV wall thickness	GRID1
LV wall thickness	WWOX
LV, Aortic root size	CCDC100
LV, aortic root size	GOSR2
LV, aortic root size	HMGA2
LV, aortic root size	LOXL1

Table 3.3 (*Continued*)

LV, aortic root size	PALMD
LV, aortic root size	PDE3A
LV, aortic root size	SMG6, SRR, TSR1
MI	LDLR
MI	PCSK9
MI	WDR12
MI	BRAP
MI	CDKN2A, CDKN2B
MI	CELSR2, PSRC1, SORT1
MI	CXCL12
MI	MIA3
MI	PHACTR1
MI	SLC5A3,MRPS6,KCNE2
Nicotine dependence	CHRNA3-NA5,CHRNB4
Nicotine dependence	CTNNA3
Nicotine dependence	FBXL17
Nicotine dependence	FTO
Nicotine dependence	NRXN1
Nicotine dependence	PBX2
Nicotine dependence	TRPC7
Nicotine dependence	VPS13A
QT interval variation	ATP1B1
QT interval variation	CNOT1,GINS3,NDRG4,..
QT interval variation	KCNJ2
QT interval variation	LIG3,RFFL
QT interval variation	LITAF,CLEC16A, SNN,..
QT interval variation	NOS1AP
QT interval variation	PLN, c6orf204, SLC35F1,..
QT interval variation	RNF207,NPHP4,CHDS,..
QT interval variation	KCNQ1/KCNH2/KCNE1
QT interval variation	SCN5A
Regular exercise	GABRG3
Regular exercise	LEPR
Regular exercise	PAPSS2
SBP	ATP2B1
SBP	CYP17A1
SBP	MTHFR
SBP	PLCD3
SBP	PLEKHA7
SBP	SH2B3
Smoking cessation	DBH

(*Continued*)

Table 3.3 (*Continued*)

Smoking initation/quantity	BDNF
Smoking initation/quantity	CDH23
Smoking initation/quantity	GRB14
Smoking initation/quantity	GRIK2
Smoking initation/quantity	GRIN2A
Smoking initation/quantity	GRIN2B
Smoking initation/quantity	GRM8
Smoking initation/quantity	NTRK2
Smoking initation/quantity	SLC1A2
Smoking initation/quantity	SLC9A9
Smoking quantity	GPSM3, AGPAT1, NOTCH4
Smoking quantity	RORB
Smoking quantity	SLCO3A1
Smoking quantity	CHRNA3-NA5, CHRNB4
Stroke	NINJ2
Stroke, ischaemic	PITX2
T2D	IGF2BP2
T2D; glucose	ADAMTS9
T2D; glucose	CDC123/CAMK1D
T2D; glucose	CDKAL1
T2D; glucose	CDKN2A, CDKN2B
T2D; glucose	FTO
T2D; glucose	HHEX, IDE
T2D; glucose	HNF1B (TCF2)
T2D; glucose	IGF2BP2
T2D; glucose	JAZF1
T2D; glucose	KCNJ11
T2D; glucose	KCNQ1
T2D; glucose	NOTCH2
T2D; glucose	PPARG
T2D; glucose	PROX1
T2D; glucose	THADA
T2D; glucose	TSPAN8, LGR5
T2D; glucose	WFS1
T2D; HOMA-B; glucose	ADCY5
T2D; HOMA-B; glucose	DGKB/TMEM195
T2D; HOMA-B; glucose	GCK
T2D; HOMA-B; glucose	MTNR1B
T2D; HOMA-B; glucose	PROX1
T2D; HOMA-B; glucose	SLC30A8
T2D; HOMA-B; glucose	TCF7L2

Table 3.3 (*Continued*)

T2D; HOMA-B; glucose; insulin	GKCR
TC	NCAN
TC	TMEM57
TC	TRIB1
TC/LDL	ABCG5
TC/LDL	APOB
TC/LDL	APOE, TOMM40
TC/LDL	CELSR2, PSRC1, SORT1
TC/LDL	DOCK7
TC/LDL	FADS2-FADS3
TC/LDL	HMGCR
TC/LDL	LDLR
Triglycerides	ANGPTL3
Triglycerides	APOA1-C3-A4-A5
Triglycerides	APOB
Triglycerides	APOE, TOMM40
Triglycerides	FADS1-FADS2-FADS3
Triglycerides	GCKR
Triglycerides	GCKR
Triglycerides	LPL
Triglycerides	MLXIPL
Triglycerides	NCAN,CILP2, PBX4
Triglycerides	PLTP
Triglycerides	TRIB1
Triglycerides	XKR6, AMAC1L2
Waist circumference	MSRA
Waist circumference	TFAP2B
Waist-hip ratio	LYPLAL1

MI – myocardial infarction; BMI – body mass index; DBP – diastolic blood pressure; HOMA IR - homoeostasis model of insulin resistance; LV – left ventricle; T2D – type 2 diabetes mellitus; SBP – systolic blood pressure.

GWA studies, showing that candidate gene selection *can* produce valid genetic targets. Examples are the genes for regulators of lipid metabolism and the genes for proteins involved in glucose transport and metabolism, that show clear association to lipids and glucose levels respectively. Perhaps the most important thing to notice is that the increased number of genes that show replicable association to CAD or CAD risk factors still account only for a small portion of the heritability of these traits. As is the case for MDD, therefore, much of the genetic regulation of CAD remains to be detected. In fact, many of the top SNPs in GWA studies (not included in Table 3.3) were in intergenic regions, and the exact pathways through which these variants exert a role on CAD risk remain to be established.

Pleiotropic Genes for MDD and CAD

In theory, the strategy to identify potential pleiotropic genes in the MDD–CAD relationship is extremely straightforward. We simply select the genes that occur in the lists of confirmed genes from the GWA studies for both traits. In practice, this is hard to do, because genetics in psychiatry is clearly lagging behind genetics in cardiology and diabetes medicine. Currently, the list of GWA-derived genes for MDD is only three: PCLO, GRM7 and TNF. The first two have not surfaced as CAD risk genes, but TNF may well be involved in the pathogenesis of the metabolic syndrome [119]. When we are willing to expand our list of MDD genes to include genes that have been successfully associated to MDD in candidate gene studies (i.e. make a cross-section of Tables 3.2 and 3.3), BDNF, ADRA2A, MTHFR and WFS1 present themselves as further potential sources of the genetic pleiotropy detected in the twin studies reviewed earlier.

CONCLUDING REMARKS

We have presented evidence from twin and family studies for a role of genetic pleiotropy in the association between MDD and CAD. The actual genetic variants that are at the base of this pleiotropy remain to be detected, but ongoing progress in gene finding through GWA studies in psychiatry will undoubtedly uncover a number of these variants in the coming decade.

Taking the concept of genetic pleiotropy to the extreme, one could argue that active attempts to prevent and treat depression in CAD patients should not have a high priority, since they would not change the subject's genotype. Such an argument could be supported by pointing to a large randomised controlled trial that targeted depressive symptoms and social isolation by behavioural therapy (ENRICHD). This did not reduce the risk for myocardial reinfarction or mortality [4], although secondary analyses may yet modify this overall picture [120]. I would like to propose a more nuanced view that regards genetic pleiotropy as an additional piece of the puzzle rather than something that should replace causal explanations. What is shown by the reviewed twin studies is that some genetic variants may influence MDD and CAD risk factors. This can occur through one of three mechanisms: (a) the genetic variants that increase the risk for MDD become part of the heritability of CAD through a causal effect of MDD on CAD risk factors (causality); (b) the genetic variants that increase the risk for CAD become part of the heritability of MDD through a direct causal effect of CAD on MDD (reverse causality); (c) the genetic variants influence shared risk factors that independently increase the risk for MDD as well as CAD (pleiotropy).

I suggest that to fully explain the MDD–CAD association we need to be willing to be open to the possibility that these three mechanisms *co-exist*. Even in the presence of true pleiotropic effects, MDD may influence CAD risk factors, and having CAD in turn may worsen the course of MDD.

REFERENCES

1. Nicholson, A., Kuper, H. and Hemingway, H. (2006) Depression as an aetiologic and prognostic factor in coronary heart disease: a meta-analysis of 6362 events among 146 538 participants in 54 observational studies. *Eur. Heart J.*, **27**, 2763–2774.

2. Alexopoulos, G.S., Meyers, B.S., Young, R.C. et al. (1997) 'Vascular depression' hypothesis. *Arch. Gen. Psychiatry*, **54**, 915–922.

3. Glassman, A.H., O'Connor, C.M., Califf, R.M. et al. (2002) Sertraline treatment of major depression in patients with acute MI or unstable angina. *JAMA*, **288**, 701–709.

4. Berkman, L.F., Blumenthal, J., Burg, M. et al. (2003) Effects of treating depression and low perceived social support on clinical events after myocardial infarction: the Enhancing Recovery in Coronary Heart Disease Patients (ENRICHD) Randomized Trial. *JAMA*, **289**, 3106–3116.

5. Ridker, P.M., Buring, J.E., Cook, N.R. and Rifai, N. (2003) C-reactive protein, the metabolic syndrome, and risk of incident cardiovascular

events: an 8-year follow-up of 14719 initially healthy American women. *Circulation*, **107**, 391–397.

6. Ridker, P.M., Rifai, N., Stampfer, M.J. and Hennekens, C.H. (2000) Plasma concentration of interleukin-6 and the risk of future myocardial infarction among apparently healthy men. *Circulation*, **101**, 1767–1772.

7. Schiepers, O.J., Wichers, M.C. and Maes, M. (2005) Cytokines and major depression. *Prog. Neuropsychopharmacol. Biol. Psychiatry*, **29**, 201–217.

8. Martin, N., Boomsma, D. and Machin, G. (1997) A twin-pronged attack on complex traits. *Nat. Genet.*, **17**, 387–392.

9. Boomsma, D., Busjahn, A. and Peltonen, L. (2002) Classical twin studies and beyond. *Nat. Rev. Genet.*, **3**, 872–882.

10. Keller, M.C., Medland, S.E., Duncan, L.E. et al. (2009) Modeling extended twin family data I: description of the Cascade model. *Twin Res. Hum. Genet.*, **12**, 8–18.

11. Boomsma, D.I., Beem, A.L., van den, B.M. et al. (2000) Netherlands twin family study of anxious depression (NETSAD). *Twin Res.*, **3**, 323–334.

12. Derks, E.M., Dolan, C.V. and Boomsma, D.I. (2006) A test of the equal environment assumption (EEA) in multivariate twin studies. *Twin Res. Hum. Genet.*, **9**, 403–411.

13. Bouchard, T.J. (1994) Genes, environment, and personality. *Science*, **264**, 1700–1701.

14. Kendler, K.S., Neale, M.C., Kessler, R.C. et al. (1994) Parental treatment and the equal environment assumption in twin studies of psychiatric illness. *Psychol. Med.*, **24**, 579–590.

15. Kendler, K.S., Neale, M.C., Kessler, R.C. et al. (1993) A test of the equal-environment assumption in twin studies of psychiatric illness. *Behav. Genet.*, **23**, 21–27.

16. Sullivan, P.F., Neale, M.C. and Kendler, K.S. (2000) Genetic epidemiology of major depression: review and meta-analysis. *Am. J. Psychiatry*, **157**, 1552–1562.

17. Mosing, M.A., Gordon, S.D., Medland, S.E. et al. (2009) Genetic and environmental influences on the co-morbidity between depression, panic disorder, agoraphobia, and social phobia: a twin study. *Depress. Anxiety*, **26**, 1004–1011.

18. Middeldorp, C.M., Birley, A.J., Cath, D.C. et al. (2005) Familial clustering of major depression and anxiety disorders in Australian and Dutch twins and siblings. *Twin Res. Hum. Genet.*, **8**, 609–615.

19. Foley, D.L., Neale, M.C. and Kendler, K.S. (1998) Reliability of a lifetime history of major depression: implications for heritability and co-morbidity. *Psychol. Med.*, **28**, 857–870.
20. Eaves, L.J., Silberg, J.L., Meyer, J.M. et al. (1997) Genetics and developmental psychopathology: 2. The main effects of genes and environment on behavioral problems in the Virginia Twin Study of Adolescent Behavioral Development. *J. Child Psychol. Psychiatry*, **38**, 965–980.
21. Eley, T.C. and Stevenson, J. (1999) Exploring the covariation between anxiety and depression symptoms: a genetic analysis of the effects of age and sex. *J. Child Psychol. Psychiatry*, **40**, 1273–1282.
22. Lau, J.Y. and Eley, T.C. (2006) Changes in genetic and environmental influences on depressive symptoms across adolescence and young adulthood. *Br. J. Psychiatry*, **189**, 422–427.
23. Boomsma, D.I., van Beijsterveldt, C.E.M., Bartels, M. and Hudziak, J.J. (2008) Genetic and environmental influence on anxious/depression: a longitudinal study in 3 to 12 year old children, in *Genetic and Environmental Influences on Developmental Psychopathology and Wellness* (ed. J.J. Hudziak), American Psychiatric Association, Washington, pp. 161–190.
24. Kendler, K.S., Gardner, C.O. and Lichtenstein, P. (2008) A developmental twin study of symptoms of anxiety and depression: evidence for genetic innovation and attenuation. *Psychol. Med.*, **38**, 1567–1575.
25. Tambs, K., Harris, J.R. and Magnus, P. (1997) Genetic and environmental contributions to the correlation between alcohol consumption and symptoms of anxiety and depression. Results from a bivariate analysis of Norwegian twin data. *Behav. Genet.*, **27**, 241–250.
26. Su, S., Miller, A.H., Snieder, H. et al. (2009) Common genetic contributions to depressive symptoms and inflammatory markers in middle-aged men: the Twins Heart Study. *Psychosom. Med.*, **71**, 152–158.
27. Gillespie, N.A., Kirk, K.M., Evans, D.M. et al. (2004) Do the genetic or environmental determinants of anxiety and depression change with age? A longitudinal study of Australian twins. *Twin Res.*, **7**, 39–53.
28. Nes, R.B., Roysamb, E., Reichborn-Kjennerud, T. et al. (2007) Symptoms of anxiety and depression in young adults: genetic and environmental influences on stability and change. *Twin Res. Hum. Genet.*, **10**, 450–461.
29. Rijsdijk, F.V., Snieder, H., Ormel, J. et al. (2003) Genetic and environmental influences on psychological distress in the population:

General Health Questionnaire analyses in UK twins. *Psychol. Med.*, **33**, 793–801.

30. Kupper, N., Willemsen, G., Riese, H. et al. (2005) Heritability of daytime ambulatory blood pressure in an extended twin design. *Hypertension*, **45**, 80–85.

31. Bak, S., Gaist, D., Sindrup, S.H. et al. (2002) Genetic liability in stroke: a long-term follow-up study of Danish twins. *Stroke*, **33**, 769–774.

32. Zdravkovic, S., Wienke, A., Pedersen, N.L. et al. (2002) Heritability of death from coronary heart disease: a 36-year follow-up of 20 966 Swedish twins. *J. Intern. Med.*, **252**, 247–254.

33. Li, M.D., Cheng, R., Ma, J.Z. and Swan, G.E. (2003) A meta-analysis of estimated genetic and environmental effects on smoking behavior in male and female adult twins. *Addiction*, **98**, 23–31.

34. Vink, J.M., Willemsen, G. and Boomsma, D.I. (2005) Heritability of smoking initiation and nicotine dependence. *Behav. Genet.*, **35**, 397–406.

35. Stubbe, J.H., Boomsma, D.I., Vink, J.M. et al. (2006) Genetic influences on exercise participation: a comparative study in adult twin samples from seven countries. *PLoS One*, **1**, e22.

36. Beunen, G. and Thomis, M. (1999) Genetic determinants of sports participation and daily physical activity. *Int. J. Obes. Relat. Metab. Disord.*, **23**, S55–S63.

37. Schousboe, K., Willemsen, G., Kyvik, K.O. et al. (2003) Sex differences in heritability of BMI: a comparative study of results from twin studies in eight countries. *Twin Res. Hum. Genet.*, **6**, 409–421.

38. Poulsen, P., Kyvik, K.O., Vaag, A. and Beck-Nielsen, H. (1999) Heritability of type II (non-insulin-dependent) diabetes mellitus and abnormal glucose tolerance – a population-based twin study. *Diabetologia*, **42**, 139–145.

39. Evans, A., van Baal, G.C., McCarron, P. et al. (2003) The genetics of coronary heart disease: the contribution of twin studies. *Twin Res. Hum. Genet.*, **6**, 432–441.

40. Beekman, M., Heijmans, B.T., Martin, N.G. et al. (2002) Heritabilities of apolipoprotein and lipid levels in three countries. *Twin Res. Hum. Genet.*, **5**, 87–97.

41. Hottenga, J.J., Whitfield, J.B., de Geus, E.J. et al. (2006) Heritability and stability of resting blood pressure in Australian twins. *Twin*, **9**, 205–209.

42. Snieder, H., van Doornen, L.J. and Boomsma, D.I. (1999) Dissecting the genetic architecture of lipids, lipoproteins, and apolipoproteins:

lessons from twin studies. *Arterioscler Thromb. Vasc. Biol.*, **19**, 2826–2834.

43. Hottenga, J.J., Boomsma, D.I., Kupper, N. et al. (2005) Heritability and stability of resting blood pressure. *Twin Res. Hum. Genet.*, **8**, 499–508.

44. Poulsen, P., Vaag, A., Kyvik, K. and Beck-Nielsen, H. (2001) Genetic versus environmental aetiology of the metabolic syndrome among male and female twins. *Diabetologia*, **44**, 537–543.

45. Liu, G.F., Riese, H., Spector, T.D. et al. (2009) Bivariate genetic modelling of the response to an oral glucose tolerance challenge: A gene x environment interaction approach. *Diabetologia*, **52**, 1048–1055.

46. Simonis-Bik, A.M.C., Eekhoff, E.M.W., Diamant, M. et al. (2008) The heritability of HbA1c and fasting blood glucose in different measurement settings. *Twin Res. Hum. Genet.*, **11**, 597–602.

47. Simonis-Bik, A.M., Eekhoff, E.M., de Moor, M.H., et al. (2009) Genetic influences on the insulin response of the beta cell to different secretagogues. *Diabetologia*, **52**, 2570–2577.

48. Retterstol, L., Eikvar, L. and Berg, K. (2003) A twin study of C-reactive protein compared to other risk factors for coronary heart disease. *Atherosclerosis*, **169**, 279–282.

49. Worns, M.A., Victor, A., Galle, P.R. and Hohler, T. (2006) Genetic and environmental contributions to plasma C-reactive protein and interleukin-6 levels – a study in twins. *Genet. Immun.*, **7**, 600–605.

50. Su, S., Snieder, H., Miller, A.H. et al. (2008) Genetic and environmental influences on systemic markers of inflammation in middle-aged male twins. *Atherosclerosis*, **200**, 213–220.

51. de Lange, M., de Geus, E.J., Kluft, C. et al. (2006) Genetic influences on fibrinogen, tissue plasminogen activator-antigen and von Willebrand factor in males and females. *Thromb. Haemost.*, **95**, 414–419.

52. Peetz, D., Victor, A., Adams, P. et al. (2004) Genetic and environmental influences on the fibrinolytic system: a twin study. *Thromb. Haemost.*, **92**, 344–351.

53. Wang, X., Ding, X., Su, S. et al. (2009) Genetic influences on heart rate variability at rest and during stress. *Psychophysiology*, **46**, 458–465.

54. Kupper, N., Willemsen, G., Boomsma, D.I. and de Geus, E.J. (2006) Heritability of indices for cardiac contractility in ambulatory recordings. *J. Cardiovasc. Electrophysiol.*, **17**, 877–883.

55. Kupper, N., Willemsen, G., Posthuma, D. et al. (2005) A genetic analysis of ambulatory cardiorespiratory coupling. *Psychophysiology*, **42**, 202–212.

56. Wu, T., Snieder, H. and Geus, E.J.C., Genetic influences on cardiovascular stress reactivity. *Neurosci. Biobehav. Rev.* (in press).

57. Neale, M.C. and Cardon, L.R. (1992) *Methodology for Genetic Studies of Twins and Families*, Kluwer, Dordrecht.

58. Scherrer, J.F., Xian, H., Bucholz, K.K. et al. (2003) A twin study of depression symptoms, hypertension, and heart disease in middle-aged men. *Psychosom. Med.*, **65**, 548–557.

59. Kendler, K.S., Gardner, C.O., Fiske, A. and Gatz, M. (2009) Major depression and coronary artery disease in the Swedish twin registry: phenotypic, genetic, and environmental sources of comorbidity. *Arch. Gen. Psychiatry*, **66**, 857–863.61.

60. Vaccarino, V., Votaw, J., Faber, T. et al. (2009) Major depression and coronary flow reserve detected by positron emission tomography. *Arch. Intern. Med.*, **169**, 1668–1676.

61. Skilton, M.R., Moulin, P., Terra, J.L. and Bonnet, F. (2007) Associations between anxiety, depression, and the metabolic syndrome. *Biol. Psychiatry*, **62**, 1251–1257.

62. Capuron, L., Su, S., Miller, A.H. et al. (2008) Depressive symptoms and metabolic syndrome: is inflammation the underlying link? *Biol. Psychiatry*, **64**, 896–900.

63. de Geus, E.J.C. and De Moor, M.H.M. (2008) A genetic perspective on the association between exercise and mental health. *Ment. Health Phys. Act*, **1**, 53–61.

64. López-León, S., Aulchenko, Y.S., Tiemeier, H., et al. (2010) Shared genetic factors in the co-occurrence of symptoms of depression and cardiovascular risk factors. *J. Affect Disord*, **122**, 247–252.

65. Vaccarino, V., Brennan, M.L., Miller, A.H. et al. (2008) Association of major depressive disorder with serum myeloperoxidase and other markers of inflammation: a twin study. *Biol. Psychiatry*, **64**, 476–483.

66. Lyons, M., Hitsman, B., Xian, H. et al. (2008) A twin study of smoking, nicotine dependence, and major depression in men. *Nicotine Tob. Res.*, **10**, 97–108.

67. McCaffery, J.M., Papandonatos, G.D., Stanton, C. et al. (2008) Depressive symptoms and cigarette smoking in twins from the National Longitudinal Study of Adolescent Health. *Health Psychol.*, **27** (Suppl. 3), S207–S215.

68. Korhonen, T., Broms, U., Varjonen, J. et al. (2007) Smoking behaviour as a predictor of depression among Finnish men and women: a prospective cohort study of adult twins. *Psychol. Med.*, **37**, 705–715.

69. Camacho, T.C., Roberts, R.E., Lazarus, N.B. et al. (1991) Physical activity and depression: evidence from the Alameda County Study. *Am. J. Epidemiol.*, **134**, 220–231.

70. Brown, W.J., Ford, J.H., Burton, N.W. et al. (2005) Prospective study of physical activity and depressive symptoms in middle-aged women. *Am. J. Prev. Med.*, **29**, 265–272.

71. Cooper-Patrick, L., Ford, D.E., Mead, L.A. et al. (1997) Exercise and depression in midlife: a prospective study. *Am. J. Publ. Health*, **87**, 670–673.

72. Farmer, M.E., Locke, B.Z., Moscicki, E.K. et al. (1988) Physical activity and depressive symptoms: the NHANES I epidemiologic follow-up study. *Am. J. Epidemiol.*, **128**, 1340–1351.

73. Kritz-Silverstein, D., Barrett-Connor, E. and Corbeau, C. (2001) Cross-sectional and prospective study of exercise and depressed mood in the elderly – The Rancho Bernardo Study. *Am. J. Epidemiol.*, **153**, 596–603.

74. Strawbridge, W.J., Deleger, S., Roberts, R.E. and Kaplan, G.A. (2002) Physical activity reduces the risk of subsequent depression for older adults. *Am. J. Epidemiol.*, **156**, 328–334.

75. van Gool, C.H., Kempen, G.I.J.M., Penninx, B.W.J.H. et al. (2003) Relationship between changes in depressive symptoms and un-healthy lifestyles in late middle aged and older persons: results from the Longitudinal Aging Study Amsterdam. *Age and Ageing*, **32**, 81–87.

76. Weyerer, S. (1992) Physical inactivity and depression in the community. Evidence from the Upper Bavarian Field Study. *Int. J. Sports Med.*, **13**, 492–496.

77. Wise, L.A., Adams-Campbell, L.L., Palmer, J.R. and Rosenberg, L. (2006) Leisure time physical activity in relation to depressive symptoms in the Black Women's Health Study. *Ann. Behav. Med.*, **32**, 68–76.

78. De Moor, M.H.M., Boomsma, D.I., Stubbe, J.H. et al. (2008) Testing causality in the association between regular exercise and symptoms of anxiety and depression. *Arch. Gen. Psychiatry*, **65**, 897–905.

79. McCaffery, J.M., Snieder, H., Dong, Y. and de Geus, E. (2007) Genetics in psychosomatic medicine: research designs and statistical approaches. *Psychosom. Med.*, **69**, 206–216.

80. López-León, S., Janssens, A.C., Gonzalez-Zuloeta Ladd, A.M. et al. (2008) Meta-analyses of genetic studies on major depressive disorder. *Mol. Psychiatry*, **13**, 772–785.

81. Sullivan, P.F., de Geus, E.J., Willemsen, G. et al. (2009) Genome-wide association for major depressive disorder: a possible role for the presynaptic protein piccolo. *Mol. Psychiatry*, **14**, 359–375.

82. Levinson, D.F. (2005) Meta-analysis in psychiatric genetics. *Curr. Psychiatry Rep.*, **7**, 143–151.

83. Lesch, K.P., Bengel, D., Heils, A. et al. (1996) Association of anxiety-related traits with a polymorphism in the serotonin transporter gene regulatory region. *Science*, **274**, 1527–1531.

84. Belmaker, R.H. and Agam, G. (2008) Major depressive disorder. *N. Engl. J. Med.*, **358**, 55–68.

85. Willis-Owen, S.A., Turri, M.G., Munafo, M.R. et al. (2005) The serotonin transporter length polymorphism, neuroticism, and depression: a comprehensive assessment of association. *Biol. Psychiatry*, **58**, 451–456.

86. Middeldorp, C.M., de Geus, E.J., Beem, A.L. et al. (2007) Family based association analyses between the serotonin transporter gene polymorphism (5-HTTLPR) and neuroticism, anxiety and depression. *Behav. Genet.*, **37**, 294–301.

87. Schinka, J.A., Busch, R.M. and Robichaux-Keene, N. (2004) A meta-analysis of the association between the serotonin transporter gene polymorphism (5-HTTLPR) and trait anxiety. *Mol. Psychiatry*, **9**, 197–202.

88. Munafo, M.R., Brown, S.M. and Hariri, A.R. (2008) Serotonin transporter (5-HTTLPR) genotype and amygdala activation: a meta-analysis. *Biol. Psychiatry*, **63**, 852–857.

89. Caspi, A., Sugden, K., Moffitt, T.E. et al. (2003) Influence of life stress on depression: moderation by a polymorphism in the 5-HTT gene. *Science*, **301**, 386–389.

90. Risch, N., Herrell, R., Lehner, T. et al. (2009) Interaction between the serotonin transporter gene (5-HTTLPR), stressful life events, and risk of depression: a meta-analysis. *JAMA*, **301**, 2462–2471.

91. Wray, N.R., James, M.R., Gordon, S.D. et al. (2009) Accurate, large-scale genotyping of 5HTTLPR and flanking single nucleotide polymorphisms in an association study of depression, anxiety, and personality measures. *Biol. Psychiatry*, **66**, 468–476.

92. Hu, X.Z., Lipsky, R.H., Zhu, G. et al. (2006) Serotonin transporter promoter gain-of-function genotypes are linked to obsessive-compulsive disorder. *Am. J. Hum. Genet.*, **78**, 815–826.

93. Levinson, D.F. (2006) The genetics of depression: a review. *Biol. Psychiatry*, **60**, 84–92.

94. Stoppel, C., Albrecht, A., Pape, H.C. and Stork, O. (2006) Genes and neurons: molecular insights to fear and anxiety. *Genes. Brain Behav.*, **5** (Suppl. 2), 34–47.

95. Muglia, P., Tozzi, F., Galwey, N.W., et al. (2010) Genome-wide association study of recurrent major depressive disorder in two European case-control cohorts. *Mol. Psychiatry*, **15**, 589–601.

96. Witkin, J.M., Marek, G.J., Johnson, B.G. and Schoepp, D.D. (2007) Metabotropic glutamate receptors in the control of mood disorders. *CNS Neurol. Disord. Drug Targets*, **6**, 87–100.

97. Bochdanovits, Z., Verhage, M., Smit, A.B. et al. (2009) Joint reanalysis of 29 correlated SNPs supports the role of PCLO/Piccolo as a causal risk factor for major depressive disorder. *Mol. Psychiatry*, **14**, 650–652.

98. Hek, K., Mulder, C.L., Luijendijk, H.J. et al. (2009) The PCLO gene and depressive disorders: replication in a population-based study. *Hum. Mol. Genet.* **19**, 731–734.

99. Cichon, S., Craddock, N., Daly, M. et al. (2009) Genomewide association studies: history, rationale, and prospects for psychiatric disorders. *Am. J. Psychiatry*, **166**, 540–556.

100. Smith, R.S. (1991) The macrophage theory of depression. *Med. Hypotheses*, **35**, 298–306.

101. Newton-Cheh, C., Johnson, T., Gateva, V., et al. Genome-wide association study identifies eight loci associated with blood pressure. *Nat. Genet.* (in press).

102. Willer, C.J., Sanna, S., Jackson, A.U. et al. (2008) Newly identified loci that influence lipid concentrations and risk of coronary artery disease. *Nat. Genet.*, **40**, 161–169.

103. McCarthy, M.I. and Zeggini, E. (2009) Genome-wide association studies in type 2 diabetes. *Curr. Diab. Rep.*, **9**, 164–171.

104. Willer, C.J., Speliotes, E.K., Loos, R.J. et al. (2009) Six new loci associated with body mass index highlight a neuronal influence on body weight regulation. *Nat. Genet.*, **41**, 25–34.

105. Arking, D.E. and Chakravarti, A. (2009) Understanding cardiovascular disease through the lens of genome-wide association studies. *Trends Genet.*, **25**, 387–394.

106. Prokopenko, I., Aulchenko, Y., Kaakinen, M. et al. (2008) Meta-analysis of genome-wide association data involving 6,100 adults of European origin identifies common variants associated with fasting glucose levels. *Diabetologia*, **51**, S11.

107. Zeggini, E., Scott, L.J., Saxena, R. et al. (2008) Meta-analysis of genome-wide association data and large-scale replication identifies additional susceptibility loci for type 2 diabetes. *Nat. Genet.*, **40**, 638–645.

108. Ikram, M.A., Seshadri, S., Bis, J.C. et al. (2009) Genomewide association studies of stroke. *N. Engl. J. Med.*, **360**, 1718–1728.

109. Aulchenko, Y.S., Ripatti, S., Lindqvist, I. et al. (2009) Loci influencing lipid levels and coronary heart disease risk in 16 European population cohorts. *Nat. Genet.*, **41**, 47–55.

110. Vasan, R.S., Glazer, N.L., Felix, J.F. et al. (2009) Genetic variants associated with cardiac structure and function: a meta-analysis and replication of genome-wide association data. *JAMA*, **302**, 168–178.

111. Freathy, R.M., Timpson, N.J., Lawlor, D.A. et al. (2008) Common variation in the FTO gene alters diabetes-related metabolic traits to the extent expected given its effect on BMI. *Diabetes*, **57**, 1419–1426.

112. Zeggini, E., Scott, L.J., Saxena, R. et al. (2008) Meta-analysis of genome-wide association data and large-scale replication identifies additional susceptibility loci for type 2 diabetes. *Nat. Genet.*, **40**, 638–645.

113. Thorleifsson, G., Walters, G.B., Gudbjartsson, D.F. et al. (2009) Genome-wide association yields new sequence variants at seven loci that associate with measures of obesity. *Nat. Genet.*, **41**, 18–24.

114. Levy, D., Ehret, G.B., Rice, K. et al. (2009) Genome-wide association study of blood pressure and hypertension. *Nat. Genet.* (in press).

115. Vink, J.M., Smit, A.B., de Geus, E.J. et al. (2009) Genome-wide association study of smoking initiation and current smoking. *Am. J. Hum. Genet.*, **84**, 367–379.

116. De Moor, M.H.M., Liu, Y.J., Boomsma, D.I., et al. Genome-wide association study of exercise behavior in Dutch and American adults. *Med. Sci. Sports Exerc.* (in press).

117. Caporaso, N., Gu, F., Chatterjee, N. et al. (2009) Genome-wide and candidate gene association study of cigarette smoking behaviors. *PLoS One*, **4**, e4653.

118. Sober, S., Org, E., Kepp, K. et al. (2009) Targeting 160 candidate genes for blood pressure regulation with a genome-wide genotyping array. *PLoS One*, **4**, e6034.

119. Sookoian, S.C., Gonzalez, C. and Pirola, C.J. (2005) Meta-analysis on the G-308A tumor necrosis factor alpha gene variant and phenotypes associated with the metabolic syndrome. *Obes. Res.*, **13**, 2122–2131.

120. Joynt, K.E. and O'Connor, C.M. (2005) Lessons from SADHART, ENRICHD, and other trials. *Psychosom. Med.*, **67**, S63–S66.

121. McCaffery, J.M., Niaura, R., Todaro, J.F. et al. (2003) Depressive symptoms and metabolic risk in adult male twins enrolled in the National Heart, Lung, and Blood Institute twin study. *Psychosom. Med.*, **65**, 490–497.

122. De Moor, M.H.M., Boomsma, D.I., Stubbe, J.H. et al. (2008) Testing causality in the association between regular exercise and symptoms of anxiety and depression. *Arch. Gen. Psychiatry*, **65**, 897–905.

CHAPTER 4

Behavioural and Psychological Mechanisms Linking Depression and Heart Disease

Roy C. Ziegelstein and Mary Kate Elfrey

Department of Medicine, Johns Hopkins Bayview Medical Center, Baltimore, MD, USA

Major depressive disorder is a global public health problem and a major cause of worldwide morbidity [1]. Of particular importance, depression is present in approximately 20% of those with heart disease [2–5]. Therefore, clinicians who provide care for patients with heart disease must be familiar with the manifestations of depression and have a heightened awareness of its symptoms. This is important because depression adversely influences the course of heart disease, and also affects all aspects of a patient's life, including family and personal relationships, education, career, sleeping and eating habits, activity and overall general health.

Other chapters of this book focus in greater detail on the epidemiology of the link between depression and heart disease, and on biological, genetic and epigenetic factors involved. In this chapter, we review the behavioural and psychological mechanisms linking depression and heart disease.

Depression and Heart Disease Edited by Alexander Glassman, Mario Maj and Norman Sartorius
© 2011 John Wiley & Sons, Ltd

BEHAVIOURAL MECHANISMS LINKING DEPRESSION AND HEART DISEASE

Patients with depression are more likely to exhibit several unhealthy behaviours or avoid other health-promoting ones than those without depression. This may be of particular relevance to heart disease, given the strong link between the health behaviours (e.g. poor diet, lack of exercise, cigarette smoking, emotional stress) and the development and progression of cardiovascular illness (Table 4.1).

Sleep Disturbance

Patients with depression are more likely to have sleep disturbances [6]. Examining the relationship of sleep disturbance and cardiovascular disease is challenging, since much of the literature on sleep and heart disease focuses on sleep apnoea rather than the sleep disturbances that are more common in the general population and among those with depression in particular. The topic is made more complicated by the fact that some cardiac conditions (e.g. heart failure) may themselves be associated with disturbed sleep as a result of problems breathing at night (i.e. orthopnoea, paroxysmal nocturnal dyspnoea) or because of the need to urinate resulting from diuretic therapy or from the improvements in renal haemodynamics and the greater ability to excrete sodium that results from nocturnal recumbency (i.e. nocturia).

Despite these challenges, several aspects of the relationship between sleep disturbance and cardiovascular disease appear clear. Sleep disturbance has been linked to cardiovascular disease mortality in the general population [7–9]. In addition, insomnia in the weeks or months prior to the event is a common complaint among those who experience a myocardial infarction, particularly among those with depression [10]. Sleep deprivation and sleep restriction are associated with autonomic hyperactivity [11], which in turn may be related to the development or worsening of various cardiovascular risk factors. Short sleep duration is associated with an increased risk of hypertension [12]. Chronic sleep deprivation is associated with changes in

Table 4.1 Behavioural mechanisms linking depression and heart disease

Mechanism	Comment	Effect on heart disease
Sleep disturbance	Common in depression; may be exacerbated by heart disease symptoms	Leads to autonomic hyperactivity which is linked to obesity, diabetes, hypertension, and the metabolic syndrome
Physical inactivity	Common in depression	Increases cardiovascular morbidity and mortality
Cigarette smoking	Individuals with depression are more likely to smoke, and depressed smokers are less likely to quit	Increases cardiovascular morbidity and mortality
Poor hygiene	Inattentiveness to self-care is more common in depression; depression is associated with decreased salivary flow and cariogenic diet. Some antidepressants cause xerostomia and gingivitis	Periodontal disease (especially gingivitis) has been associated with increased cardiovascular morbidity and mortality
Adherence to treatment	Patients with depression are less likely to adhere to medical therapy and risk reducing behaviours	Poor adherence to medical therapy is associated with increased cardiovascular morbidity and mortality

levels of leptin and ghrelin, hormones that are important in appetite regulation [13]. As a consequence of these and other changes, sleep deprivation has been linked with obesity, diabetes and the metabolic syndrome [13].

Physical Inactivity

Depression is associated with an increased risk of physical inactivity [14, 15]. This is particularly important with respect to cardiovascular disease, given the association of low physical activity levels and adverse cardiovascular health outcomes [16]. Low levels of physical activity are an independent risk factor for the development of cardiovascular disease [17] and, in contrast, regular physical activity is associated with decreased mortality from heart disease [18]. Physical inactivity and depression display a complex, bidirectional relationship. Depression leads to physical inactivity and physical inactivity exacerbates depression [19].

In a group of over 1000 outpatients with stable cardiovascular disease, the association between depressive symptoms and an increased risk of cardiovascular events was found to be largely explained by physical inactivity [20]. Increased physical activity can improve symptoms of depression [21]. The relationship of physical inactivity and depression is particularly important given the evidence that physical inactivity is associated with the development or worsening of many cardiac risk factors (e.g. obesity, diabetes mellitus, hyperlipidaemia) and that regular physical activity reduces the risk of heart disease and mortality [22].

Regular physical activity is associated with improvements in blood pressure, glycaemic control and lipid levels [22]. In a recent multicentre, randomised controlled trial of usual care plus aerobic exercise training compared with usual care alone among more than 2000 outpatients with systolic heart failure, exercise training resulted in significant reductions in all-cause mortality or hospitalisation and in cardiovascular mortality or heart failure hospitalisation after adjustment for highly prognostic baseline characteristics [23]. Exercise training also resulted in improvements in self-reported health status in these patients that were sustained over more than 2 years [24]. In addition to the benefits of exercise on cardiovascular risk factors and cardiac outcomes, the effect of exercise on depression itself must be considered. Although the evidence is limited and additional research on the topic is needed, exercise may be either an alternative or adjunctive treatment for depression [25].

Cigarette Smoking

Several observations point to a link between cigarette smoking and depression that may be a mechanism that makes depressed patients more likely to develop heart disease. Individuals with major depression are more likely to smoke cigarettes than the general population [26–28]. In fact, smoking rates among those with depression are about twice that of the general population [29]. Smokers are more likely to experience depression in their lifetime than those who have never smoked [29]. Depressed smokers are less likely to quit than smokers who do not suffer with depression [29]. This may be because it is well recognised that smoking cessation often precipitates depression [30, 31].

Although the basic cellular mechanisms that link smoking and depression are incompletely understood, neuronal nicotinic acetyl-choline receptors (nAChRs) are felt to be important in this relation-ship. Nicotine exerts its effect by binding to nAChRs, which are widely distributed in the brain [32]. The intravenous administration of nicotine produces a sense of euphoria that is similar to that of cocaine [29]. Nicotine possesses antidepressant-like activity in the central nervous system largely mediated by stimulation of nAChRs, which increases the release of dopamine, noradrenaline and serotonin in the brain [32]. The antidepressant-like activity of cigarette smoke also derives from chemicals other than nicotine, which act as mono-amine oxidase inhibitors [31–33]. Thus, cigarette smoke decreases the activity of monoamine oxidase in the brain, which would, in turn, increase concentrations of dopamine, norepinephrine and serotonin in the central nervous system.

In addition to the possible mood-elevating effects of cigarette smoking that may make depressed individuals more likely to smoke, depressed individuals may experience greater reward from smoking as a result of a dysfunctional dopaminergic brain reward system. The notion that depression may be associated with greater reward from smoking comes from a study that showed that depressed subjects were more sensitive to activation of the dopaminergic brain reward system by d-amphetamine, which releases dopamine in the central nervous system [34].

Since smoking is a well-known risk factor for cardiac disease, the impact of the strong link between cigarette smoking and depression on health is clear. And unfortunately, depressive symptoms during hospitalisations for cardiac disease are independently associated with rapid relapse to smoking after discharge and lower rates of smoking cessation at long-term follow-up [35–37].

Poor Hygiene

Poor attention to self-care is often a problem among those with major depressive disorder. In the most severe cases, those with depression may become inattentive to their personal hygiene. One aspect of this relationship that deserves special attention with respect to cardiovascular disease is the association of depression and periodontal disease. In addition to poor oral hygiene, several other factors may lead to an increased prevalence of periodontal disease in depressed patients. Stress and depression are associated with chronic inflammation that can result in gingivitis and periodontal disease [38]. Depression is also associated with reduced salivary flow and with a diet that may lead to dental caries and gingivitis [39]. In addition, many antidepressants can produce xerostomia, sialadenitis, dysgeusia and gingivitis [40]. These factors, coupled with poor oral hygiene, lead to a more exuberant oral biofilm and diminished resistance of the periodontium to inflammation [41, 42]. The link between depression and periodontal disease is especially important given the evidence that periodontal disease is associated with cardiovascular disease, and that this association persists even after adjusting for other known cardiovascular risk factors. This may be because periodontitis is associated with systemic inflammation, including increased systemic concentrations of C-reactive protein, fibrinogen and pro-inflammatory cytokines [43].

Poor Adherence to Treatment

Almost half of all medical patients in the United States do not adhere to their physicians' recommendations for prevention or treatment of medical conditions [44]. Among those with heart disease, poor adherence is typically manifested by not taking medications correctly, not following a proper diet, not engaging in recommended exercise regimens or not participating in (or dropping out from) cardiac rehabilitation programmes. Those who are not good adherers may also cancel or miss appointments and persist in unhealthy lifestyles or behaviours that jeopardise their health. This is important because the consequences often result in exacerbation of illness, inaccurate diagnoses and patient and physician frustration. There is growing evidence that poor adherence has significant negative effects on treatment outcomes [45, 46].

Many factors affect patients' adherence to medical treatment regimens. Among these are the complexity of the medical regimen itself, the cost of the medical regimen, medication side effects and the availability of health insurance. In addition, depression is associated with poor adherence to medical treatment regimens in many chronic illnesses, including heart disease. In fact, the odds are three times greater that depressed patients will not adhere to medical treatment recommendations than those without depression [44].

Among those with heart disease, one early study [47] assessed adherence to aspirin (using an electronic medication-monitoring device that records the date and time each pill is removed from a medication packet) in 55 patients undergoing elective coronary angiography, 10 of whom had major depressive disorder based on a structured clinical interview. In these patients, major depression was associated with poor adherence to daily aspirin. Similar findings have been reported in several other studies. In one larger study that also assessed adherence to aspirin using an electronic-monitoring device (located in the pill bottle cap), 165 patients with an acute coronary syndrome were assessed for depressive symptoms using the Beck Depression Inventory (BDI) both at baseline and again 3 months later [48]. A similar percentage (about 10%) of patients who were never depressed and whose depressive symptoms remitted in the 3-month period took aspirin 75% of the time or less (i.e. were poor adherers to aspirin). However, a significantly greater percentage of those with persistent depression adhered poorly to aspirin (42.1%). In another study, compared with a group of stable outpatients with coronary artery disease but without depression, those with major depressive disorder based on a structured clinical interview reported significantly more often that they did not take their medications as prescribed, that they forgot to take their medications, or that they skipped their medications [49]. There is some evidence that among patients with an acute coronary syndrome, improvement in depression is associated with improvement in adherence. In particular, medication adherence improves in patients who experience complete remission of depression [50].

One study assessed the relation between depression during hospitalisation for a heart attack and engagement in cardiac risk-modifying behaviours and adherence to medications 4 months later. Patients with symptoms of at least mild-to-moderate depression (based on BDI) or with major depression and/or dysthymia (based on a structured clinical interview for depression) during the initial hospitalisation reported lower adherence to a low-fat diet, regular exercise, reducing stress and increasing social support when interviewed by telephone 4 months later [51]. Compared with those without depression, those with major depression and/or dysthymia during the initial hospitalisation reported taking medications as prescribed less often 4 months later.

In addition to these studies that were mostly in patients with coronary artery disease, the relationship between depression and poor adherence has also been demonstrated in other heart disease populations. For example, among patients with heart failure, depression has been shown to be associated with poorer adherence to dietary recommendations [52] and self-reported difficulty taking medications [53]. Among patients attending a general outpatient cardiology clinic, higher levels of depressive symptoms were associated with greater self-reported medication non-adherence [54]. Depression is also associated with higher rates of dropout from cardiac rehabilitation programmes before the recommended course of treatment has been completed [55–58].

Depression was also shown to affect adherence to warfarin anticoagulation among patients who underwent aortic valve replacement surgery with a mechanical prosthesis [59]. In this study, adherence was assessed by supplying warfarin in pill bottles with a microprocessor in the cap that registered the time of opening the bottle. Nondepressed patients adhered to their medical regimen significantly more often than those with depression (97.0% vs. 86.2%) and also attended the anticoagulation clinic as recommended significantly more often (96.7% vs. 53.1%).

PSYCHOLOGICAL MECHANISMS LINKING DEPRESSION AND HEART DISEASE

Attitudes About the Treatment of Cardiac Disease

Individuals with cardiovascular disease who take their medications as prescribed (so-called 'good adherers') fare better than those who do not. This finding does not seem surprising, since so many drug treatments (e.g. aspirin, lipid-lowering medications and beta blockers) reduce morbidity and mortality in patients with heart disease. What may be surprising is the number of studies that have shown that 'good adherers' with cardiovascular disease fare better even when they adhere well to a regimen of inactive placebo tablets (Table 4.2).

In the Coronary Drug Project Research Group study [45], the Beta-Blocker Heart Attack Trial [46], the Canadian Amiodarone Myocardial Infarction Arrhythmia Trial [60] and the Candesartan in Heart failure: Assessment of Reduction in Mortality and morbidity trial [61], those who were considered 'good adherers' had an almost identically lower mortality in both the active treatment and placebo groups. In a meta-analysis of eight studies involving 19 633 subjects that examined the association of mortality and adherence to either active medical therapy or to placebo, Simpson et al. [62] found that, compared with poor adherence to placebo, good adherence to placebo was associated with a strikingly lower mortality (OR 0.56; 95% CI 0.43, 0.74). The relationship between adherence and mortality in the placebo arm was virtually identical in the active treatment arm of those studies in which beneficial drug therapy was studied (OR 0.55; 95% CI 0.49, 0.62).

These findings suggest that beliefs and attitudes towards treatment may play an important role in treatment response, and that conditions associated with negative attitudes towards treatment may be associated with poorer response. Depression may be one such condition that is associated with negative attitudes towards treatment. Chao et al. [63] surveyed individuals with type 2 diabetes to assess depressive symptoms, diabetes-related health beliefs and diabetes medication adherence. Based on the results from 445 individuals, the authors developed a structural equation model to address whether diabetes-related health beliefs mediate the relationship between depressive symptoms and adherence. In this study, depressive symptoms were

Table 4.2 Psychological mechanisms linking depression and heart disease

Mechanism	Comment	Effect on heart disease
Attitudes about treatment	Depression may be associated with negative attitudes toward treatment. Individuals with depression may perceive more, and have greater concern about, medication side effects	Attitudes about treatment appear important to therapeutic effect; even poor adherers to placebo in cardiovascular disease trials have increased mortality
Social isolation	Depression is associated with less social support and greater social isolation	Decreased social support and social isolation are associated with increased cardiovascular morbidity and mortality
Cardiovascular stress response	Studies are inconsistent. Some show that depression is associated with heightened, and some with attenuated, cardiovascular reactivity to physiological stress; both may actually be the case (see text)	Autonomic hyperactivity at baseline and in response to stressors may increase cardiovascular risk
Self-efficacy	Depression is often associated with low self-efficacy	Low self-efficacy is associated with greater symptom burden and physical limitation; with worse quality of life; with poor adherence; and possibly with increased cardiovascular morbidity and mortality

associated with poor adherence, as expected. Of note, this association was partially explained by patients' beliefs about their medications. In particular, the authors noted that patients with comorbid diabetes and depression might perceive more side effects from their medications, have greater concern about potential side effects or perceive more inconvenience regarding taking medication than those patients with diabetes who are not depressed. This may also be the case in patients with cardiovascular disease. Bane et al. [54] performed a multidimensional assessment of 122 outpatients with cardiovascular disease that included a measure of depression (the Center for Epidemiological Studies Depression Scale, CES-D), beliefs about medications (the Beliefs about Medicines Questionnaire, BMQ) and self-reported medication adherence. Higher scores on the CES-D (more depressive symptoms) and strong concern scores about potential adverse effects of medications on the BMQ were both associated with self-reported non-adherence. Of note, high scores on the CES-D were associated with high concern scores on the BMQ, suggesting that patients with cardiovascular disease who have high levels of depressive symptoms also have strong concerns about their medications. These findings suggest that an individual's beliefs and attitudes about medical treatment may be important in determining his/her response to therapy. Those individuals with depression may be more likely to have concerns about treatment, and their negative beliefs and attitudes may have important effects on multiple outcomes, including mortality.

Social Isolation

Individuals with depression are often socially withdrawn or isolated. It has been shown that patients with heart disease who are depressed have less social support [64], and that social isolation or poor social support is associated with increased mortality in heart disease patients [65–68]. Indeed, studies in the 1980s and 1990s showed that individuals recovering from a myocardial infarction who are either socially isolated [69] or live alone [70] are at increased risk of death. Although certainly many of those who live alone are not depressed and may not be socially isolated, living alone is often considered a proxy for social isolation and poor social support [71]. The observation that living alone is associated with higher mortality in patients having a heart attack was confirmed more recently [71] in a study of 880 patients with a myocardial infarction. The 164 patients who lived alone (18.6%) had a 1.6-fold greater mortality risk than those who were living with others; the mortality risk was twofold higher in men who lived alone. Of note, men who live alone are more likely to be depressed than women who live alone [72].

The health risks of social isolation or lack of social support may be particularly high for individuals who are depressed. Depressed individuals may be particularly dependent on encouragement from others, since they may lack the motivation to engage in healthy behaviours and to avoid unhealthy ones. There are certainly many reasons why living alone may confer risk in heart disease. One area that has received attention is the association of living alone and the time from the onset of symptoms to the time an individual seeks medical attention. Delayed presentations are associated with increased myocardial injury and infarct size [73] and higher mortality [74]. Moreover, there is an inverse relationship between time to presentation from symptom onset and the benefit of reperfusion therapy, when an intervention is given to open an occluded coronary artery by drug therapy (e.g. thrombolytic treatment) [74, 75] or device therapy (e.g. percutaneous coronary intervention) [76, 77]. Individuals who live alone may not benefit from the encouragement to seek care that those who live with others might have. It has been suggested that living alone may be particularly risky for men because men are more reliant on the encouragement of their spouses to seek medical attention for symptoms of heart disease [71].

The findings above, therefore, suggest that clinicians who make recommendations to patients recovering from a heart attack should be aware that low levels of social support and social isolation are particularly common among depressed individuals and that high levels of social support appear to protect patients from some of the negative effects of depression [78].

Response to Physiological Stress

Stressful life experiences are common in everyday life. Some have hypothesised that depression may be associated with a heightened response to physiological stress, and that exaggerated cardiovascular reactivity to stress may be at least partially responsible for the increased morbidity and mortality associated with depression in heart disease patients.

There is little consistency in the literature on this topic that permits support for this hypothesis. Some authors have found that depression is associated with an exaggerated stress response [79], others have reported no consistent association [80], and still others have found that those with major depressive disorder have a blunted cardiovascular stress response. Indeed, in a recent study, depressed individuals demonstrated significantly less reactivity of systolic blood pressure, heart rate and cardiac output during stress-producing tasks (e.g. preparing and delivering a speech on a stress-producing topic such as defending themselves against a traffic ticket) than healthy control subjects, despite appraising these tasks as more stressful [81]. Similarly, an inverse relationship between scores on the BDI (the higher the scores, the more depressive symptoms) and cardiovascular reactivity was documented in a study of patients with established coronary artery disease who were subjected to psychological stress testing by public speaking about a real-life problem [82].

The observation that individuals with depression may have an attenuated cardiovascular stress response is particularly curious, since there is also evidence of sympathetic nervous system activation in patients with major depression [83], marked by increased plasma noradrenaline [84, 85] and cortisol [86]. In addition, there is some evidence that depression is associated with an exaggerated noradrenaline response to acute stress [87, 88]. Decreased adrenergic receptor sensitivity [89, 90] or number [90–93] might explain the attenuated cardiovascular stress response in those with major depression. Individuals with depression may also represent a heterogeneous group, with some individuals demonstrating an increased stress response and others demonstrating either a normal or attenuated response. This possibility is supported by the finding that whole body and cardiac sympathetic activity is extraordinarily high in some individuals with major depressive disorder while in others it is very low [94]. This finding may be unique to those with major depression, since it has not been reported in any other condition. Thus, there may be some individuals with major depression who have exaggerated cardiovascular reactivity to acute physiological stress, and may therefore be at increased cardiovascular risk. However, more research is needed in this area to clarify this possibility.

Self-Efficacy

Self-efficacy describes an individual's self-confidence in his/her ability to accomplish a particular task or behaviour. Self-efficacy is an important construct to consider when one examines the psychological mechanisms linking depression and heart disease, since it influences an individual's engagement in behaviour and lifestyle changes that may be critical to improving cardiovascular risk. Many studies on individuals with chronic illness show that depression is often associated with low self-efficacy [95–97]. If a depressed patient with heart disease had low self-efficacy, he/she would lack confidence in his/her ability to engage in certain healthy behaviours (e.g. exercising or following a proper diet) or avoid unhealthy ones (e.g. smoking cigarettes). It is thought that this lack of confidence, in turn, even independent of depressed mood, would negatively influence the individual's actual performance of those behaviours, and ultimately negatively affect health outcomes.

Among patients with coronary artery disease, self-efficacy has been shown to predict physical function, social function and family function [98]. In the Heart and Soul Study, self-efficacy was assessed in a group of over 1000 outpatients with stable coronary heart disease. In one report from this cohort [99], low 'cardiac self-efficacy' (i.e. low levels of confidence in the ability to take care of health) independently predicted greater symptom burden, greater physical limitation, worse quality of life, and worse overall health. Not surprisingly, low self-efficacy was associated with depressive symptoms, and depressive symptoms partially mediated the effect of self-efficacy on health status. Importantly, though, low self-efficacy was independently associated with poor health status. In another report from the Heart and Soul Study, lower self-efficacy predicted subsequent heart failure hospitalisation and all-cause mortality, although this was explained by worse baseline cardiac function [100]. Low self-efficacy is associated with poor adherence behaviour in patients with heart failure [101].

Much of the interest in self-efficacy comes from the fact that it is modifiable. Self-efficacy-enhancing interventions have been shown to improve cardiac patients' self-efficacy and thereby improve cardiac health outcomes [102]. In addition, strategies that target self-efficacy in at-risk populations have shown that they can improve physical activity and cardiorespiratory fitness in obese, sedentary women [103] and enhance readiness to quit among women who smoke [104]. One problem with targeting self-efficacy in depressed heart disease patients is that depressive symptoms reduce the effects of self-efficacy-enhancing interventions [105, 106]. Nevertheless, self-efficacy remains an important target for interventions that might affect the relationship between depression and cardiovascular morbidity and mortality.

CONCLUSIONS

The relationship between depression and heart disease is now well-established. This relationship is important, both because of the high prevalence of these two conditions, and because of their health burden, especially when they occur together. This chapter reviewed many of the behavioural and psychological mechanisms involved in this relationship. Of the behavioural mechanisms, this chapter focused on the greater difficulty engaging in healthy behaviours (e.g. good sleep habits, physical activity, good hygiene, adherence to medical therapy and to recommendations intended to reduce cardiac risk, completion of recommended cardiac rehabilitation programmes) and on the greater likelihood of engaging in unhealthy ones (e.g. cigarette smoking, poor diet). Of the psychological mechanisms, this chapter focused on low self-efficacy, social isolation, poor social support, response to physiological stress, and greater concerns and negative beliefs and attitudes about cardiac treatment regimens.

The goal of this chapter was not only to review the link between behavioural and psychological mechanisms and heart disease, but also to leave clinicians with 'take home points' that might help them as they provide care for their patients with comorbid depression and heart disease. In this regard, the following recommendations are offered:

Sleep. Ask your patients about their sleep habits. Treating depression may improve sleep duration and allow for greater periods of uninterrupted sleep. Ask about why patients are awakening, and see if changes in treatment or the timing of medications might decrease the need to awaken during the night to pass urine or because of breathlessness.

Physical activity. Strongly encourage your patients to exercise at home and to become involved (and stay involved) in structured exercise programmes. Treating depression may improve physical activity, and greater involvement in exercise may improve symptoms of depression.

Cigarette smoking. Ask every patient whether he/she smokes at every visit and counsel patients about smoking cessation if appropriate. Every clinician should become familiar with medications that help patients quit, and should offer patients specific advice on how to quit and/or in setting a quit date.

Oral hygiene. Enquire about oral hygiene habits and examine the mouth.

Medication adherence. Specifically address the issue of medication adherence with every patient and try to decrease barriers to adherence if possible. Clinicians should anticipate greater problems with adherence among their patients who are depressed. Simplifying medication regimens, eliminating medications that are not absolutely necessary, and prescribing low-cost alternatives may be helpful in specific circumstances.

Attitudes and beliefs about cardiac treatment regimens. Anticipate the possibility that patients with depression may have greater levels of concern and more negative attitudes and beliefs about medical treatment regimens. Discuss the importance of each medication, what the goals of treatment are, and how the patient's particular health goals are more likely to be achieved by adhering to a particular medical treatment.

Social isolation. Encourage patients to socialise with family and friends; offer to engage family and friends on behalf of the patient, encourage the patient to participate in group activities that may be appropriate and desirable to the individual (sports clubs, hobbies, religious groups).

Self-efficacy. Enquire about your patient's confidence that he or she can accomplish a given task or behaviour (e.g. participation in a cardiac rehabilitation programme, stopping smoking, following a proper diet). If the patient's confidence is low, consider specific counselling that might enhance self efficacy.

ACKNOWLEDGEMENTS AND DISCLAIMER

Dr Ziegelstein is supported by the grant R24AT004641 from the National Center for Complementary and Alternative Medicine and by the Miller Family Scholar Program of the Johns Hopkins Center for Innovative Medicine. The content of this chapter is solely the responsibility of the authors and does not necessarily represent the official views of the National Center for Complementary and Alternative Medicine or the National Institutes of Health.

REFERENCES

1. Moussavi, S., Chatterji, S., Verdes, E. et al. (2007) Depression, chronic diseases, and decrements in health: results from the World Health Surveys. *Lancet*, **370**, 851–858.
2. Thombs, B.D., Bass, E.B., Ford, D.E. et al. (2006) Prevalence of depression in survivors of acute myocardial infarction. *J. Gen. Intern. Med.*, **21**, 30–38.
3. Rudisch, B. and Nemeroff, C.B. (2003) Epidemiology of comorbid coronary artery disease and depression. *Biol. Psychiatry*, **54**, 227–240.
4. Rutledge, T., Reis, V.A., Linke, S.E. et al. (2006) Depression in heart failure: a meta-analytic review of prevalence, intervention effects, and associations with clinical outcomes. *J. Am. Coll. Cardiol.*, **48**, 1527–1537.
5. Bush, D.E., Ziegelstein, R.C., Tayback, M. et al. (2001) Even minimal symptoms of depression increase mortality risk after acute myocardial infarction. *Am. J. Cardiol.*, **88**, 337–341.
6. Ford, D. and Cooper-Patrick, L. (2001) Sleep disturbances and mood disorders: an epidemiologic perspective. *Depress. Anxiety*, **14**, 3–6.
7. Mallon, L., Broman, J.-E. and Hetta, J. (2002) Sleep complaints predict coronary artery disease mortality in males: a 12-year follow-up study of a middle-aged Swedish population. *J. Intern. Med.*, **251**, 207–216.
8. Nicholson, A., Fuhrer, R. and Marmot, M. (2005) Psychological distress as a predictor of CHD events in men: the effect of persistence and components of risk. *Psychosom. Med.*, **67**, 522–530.

9. Eaker, E.D., Pinsky, J. and Castelli, W.P. (1992) Myocardial infarction and coronary death among women: psychosocial predictors from a 20-year follow-up of women in the Framingham Study. *Am. J. Epidemiol.*, **135,** 854–864.

10. Carney, R.M., Freedland, K.E. and Jaffe, A.S. (1990) Insomnia and depression prior to myocardial infarction. *Psychosom. Med.*, **52,** 603–609.

11. Meerlo, P., Sgoifo, A. and Suchecki, D. (2008) Restricted and disrupted sleep: effects on autonomic function, neuroendocrine stress systems and stress responsivity. *Sleep Med. Rev.*, **12,** 197–210.

12. Gangwisch, J.E., Heymsfield, S.B., Boden-Albala, B. et al. (2006) Short sleep duration as a risk factor for hypertension: analyses of the first National Health and Nutrition Examination Survey. *Hypertension*, **47,** 833–839.

13. Van Cauter, E., Spiegel, K., Tasali, E. and Leproult, R. (2008) Metabolic consequences of sleep and sleep loss. *Sleep Med.*, **9,** S23–S28.

14. Koopmans, B., Pouwer, F., de Bie, R.A. et al. (2009) Depressive symptoms are associated with physical inactivity in patients with type 2 diabetes. *Fam. Pract.*, **26,** 171–173.

15. Kamphuis, M.H., Geerlings, M.I., Tijhuis, M.A.R. et al. (2007) Physical inactivity, depression, and risk of cardiovascular mortality. *Med. Sci. Sports Exerc.*, **39,** 1693–1699.

16. Mozaffarian, D., Furberg, C.D., Psaty, B.M. and Siscovick, D. (2008) Physical activity and incidence of atrial fibrillation in older adults: the Cardiovascular Health Study. *Circulation*, **118,** 800–807.

17. Powell, K.E., Thompson, P.D., Caspersen, C.J. and Kendrick, J.S. (1987) Physical activity and the incidence of coronary heart disease. *Annu. Rev. Publ. Health*, **8,** 253–287.

18. Haapanen-Niemi, N., Miilunpalo, S., Pasanen, M. et al. (2000) Body mass index, physical inactivity and low level of physical fitness as determinants of all-cause and cardiovascular disease mortality: 16 year follow-up of middle-aged and elderly men and women. *Int. J. Obes. Relat. Metab. Disord.*, **24,** 1465–1474.

19. Weyerer, S. and Kupfer, B. (1994) Physical exercise and psychological health. *Sports Med.*, **17,** 108–116.

20. Whooley, M.A., De Jonge, P., Vittinghoff, E. et al. (2008) Depressive symptoms, health behaviors, and risk of cardiovascular events in patients with coronary heart disease. *JAMA*, **300,** 2379–2388.

21. Blumenthal, J.A., Babyak, M.A., Doraiswamy, P.M. et al. (2007) Exercise and pharmacotherapy in the treatment of major depressive disorder. *Psychosom. Med.*, **69,** 587–596.

22. Warburton, D.E., Nicol, C.W. and Bredin, S.S. (2006) Health benefits of physical activity: the evidence. *CMAJ*, **174**, 801–809.

23. O'Connor, C.M., Whellan, D.J., Lee, K.L. et al. (2009) Efficacy and safety of exercise training in patients with chronic heart failure: HF-ACTION randomized controlled trial. *JAMA*, **301**, 1439–1450.

24. Flynn, K.E., Piña, I.L., Whellan, D.J. et al. (2009) Effects of exercise training on health status in patients with chronic heart failure: HF-ACTION randomized controlled trial. *JAMA*, **301**, 1451–1459.

25. Mead, G.E., Morley, W., Campbell, P. et al. (2009) Exercise for depression. *Cochrane Database Syst. Rev.*, **3**, CD004366.

26. Hughes, J.R., Hatsukami, D.K., Mitchell, J.E. and Dahlgreen, L.A. (1986) Prevalence of smoking among psychiatric outpatients. *Am. J. Psychiatry*, **143**, 993–997.

27. Laje, R.P., Berman, J.A. and Glassman, A.H. (2001) Depression and nicotine: preclinical and clinical evidence for common mechanisms. *Curr. Psychiatry Rep.*, **3**, 470–474.

28. Paperwalla, K.N., Levin, T.T., Weiner, J. and Saravay, S.M. (2004) Smoking and depression. *Med. Clin. North Am.*, **88**, 1483–1494.

29. Glassman, A.H., Helzer, J.E. and Covey, L.S. (1990) Smoking, smoking cessation, and major depression. *JAMA*, **264**, 1546–1549.

30. Covey, L.S., Glassman, A.H. and Stetner, F. (1997) Major depression following smoking cessation. *Am. J. Psychiatry*, **154**, 263–265.

31. Glassman, A.H., Covey, L.S., Stetner, F. and Rivelli, S. (2001) Smoking cessation and the course of major depression: a follow-up study. *Lancet*, **357**, 1929–1932.

32. Quattrocki, E., Baird, A. and Yurgelun-Todd, D. (2000) Biological aspects of the link between smoking and depression. *Harv. Rev. Psychiatry*, **8**, 99–110.

33. Fowler, J.S., Volkow, N.D., Wang, G.J. et al. (1996) Brain monoamine oxidase A inhibition in cigarette smokers. *Proc. Natl. Acad. Sci.*, **93**, 14065–14069.

34. Cardenas, L., Tremblay, L.K., Naranjo, C.A. et al. (2002) Brain reward system activity in major depression and comorbid nicotine dependence. *J. Pharmacol. Exp. Ther.*, **302**, 1265–1271.

35. Thorndike, A., Regan, S., McKool, K. et al. (2008) Depressive symptoms and smoking cessation after hospitalization for cardiovascular disease. *Arch. Intern. Med.*, **168**, 186–191.

36. Dawood, N., Vaccarino, V., Reid, K.J. et al. (2008) Predictor of smoking cessation after a myocardial infarction: the role of institutional smoking

cessation programs in improving success. *Arch. Intern. Med.*, **168,** 1961–1967.

37. Perez, G.H., Nicolau, J.C., Romano, B.W. and Laranjeira, R. (2008) Depression: a predictor of smoking relapse in a 6-month follow-up after hospitalization for acute coronary syndrome. *Eur. J. Cardiovasc. Prev. Rehabil.*, **15,** 89–94.

38. Hilgert, J.B., Hugo, F.N., Bandeira, D.R. and Bozzetti, M.C. (2006) Stress, cortisol, and periodontitis in a population aged 50 years and over. *J. Dent. Res.*, **85,** 324–328.

39. Friedlander, A.H. and West, L.J. (1991) Dental management of the patient with major depression. *Oral Surg. Oral Med. Oral Pathol.*, **71,** 573–578.

40. Friedlander, A.H. and Mahler, M.E. (2001) Major depressive disorder. Psychopathology, medical management and dental implications. *J. Am. Dent. Assoc.*, **132,** 629–638.

41. Peruzzo, D.C., Benatti, B.B., Ambrosano, G.M. et al. (2007) A systematic review of stress and psychological factors as possible risk factors for periodontal disease. *J. Periodontol.*, **78,** 1491–1504.

42. Rosania, A.E., Low, K.G., McCormick, C.M. and Rosania, D.A. (2009) Stress, depression, cortisol, and periodontal disease. *J. Periodontol.*, **80,** 260–266.

43. Scannapieco, F.A., Bush, R.B. and Paju, S. (2003) Associations between periodontal disease and risk for atherosclerosis, cardiovascular disease, and stroke. A systematic review. *Ann. Periodontol.*, **8,** 38–53.

44. DiMatteo, M.R., Lepper, H.S. and Croghan, T.W. (2000) Depression is a risk factor for noncompliance with medical treatment: meta-analysis of the effects of anxiety and depression on patient adherence. *Arch. Intern. Med.*, **160,** 2101–2107.

45. Coronary Drug Project Research Group (1980) Influence of adherence to treatment and response of cholesterol on mortality in the coronary drug project. *N. Engl. J. Med.*, **303,** 1038–1041.

46. Horwitz, R.I., Viscoli, C.M. and Berkman, L. (1990) Treatment adherence and risk of death after a myocardial infarction. *Lancet*, **336,** 542–545.

47. Carney, R.M., Freedland, K.E., Eisen, S.A. et al. (1995) Major depression and medication adherence in elderly patients with coronary artery disease. *Health Psychol.*, **14,** 88–90.

48. Rieckmann, N., Kronish, I.M., Haas, D. et al. (2006) Persistent depressive symptoms lower aspirin adherence after acute coronary syndromes. *Am. Heart J.*, **152,** 922–927.

49. Gehi, A., Haas, D., Pipkin, S. and Whooley, M.A. (2005) Depression and medication adherence in outpatients with coronary heart disease; findings from the Heart and Soul Study. *Arch. Intern. Med.*, **165**, 2508–2513.

50. Glassman, A.H., Bigger, J.T. Jr. and Gaffney, M. (2009) Psychiatric characteristics associated with long-term mortality among 361 patients having an acute coronary syndrome and major depression: seven-year follow-up of SADHART participants. *Arch. Gen. Psychiatry*, **66**, 1022–1029.

51. Ziegelstein, R.C., Fauerbach, J.A., Stevens, S.S. et al. (2000) Patients with depression are less likely to follow recommendations to reduce cardiac risk during recovery from a myocardial infarction. *Arch. Intern. Med.*, **160**, 1818–1823.

52. Luyster, F.S., Hughes, J.W. and Gunstad, J. (2009) Depression and anxiety symptoms are associated with reduced dietary adherence in heart failure patients treated with an implantable cardioverter defibrillator. *J. Cardiovasc. Nurs.*, **24**, 10–17.

53. Morgan, A.L., Masoudi, F.A., Havranek, E.P. et al. (2006) Difficulty taking medications, depression, and health status in heart failure patients. *J. Cardiac Failure*, **12**, 54–60.

54. Bane, C., Hughes, C.M. and McElnay, J.C. (2006) The impact of depressive symptoms and psychosocial factors on medication adherence in cardiovascular disease. *Patient Educ. Couns.*, **60**, 187–193.

55. Casey, E., Hughes, J.W., Waechter, D. et al. (2008) Depression predicts failure to complete phase-II cardiac rehabilitation. *J. Behav. Med.*, **31**, 421–431.

56. Caulin-Glaser, T., Maciejewski, P.K., Snow, R. et al. (2007) Depressive symptoms and sex affect completion rates and clinical outcomes in cardiac rehabilitation. *Prev. Cardiol.*, **10**, 15–21.

57. Glazer, K.M., Emery, C.F., Frid, D.J. and Banyasz, R.E. (2002) Psychological predictors of adherence and outcomes among patients in cardiac rehabilitation. *J. Cardiopulm. Rehabil.*, **22**, 40–46.

58. Blumenthal, J.A., Williams, R.S., Wallace, A.G. et al. (1982) Physiological and psychological variables predict compliance to prescribed exercise therapy in patients recovering from myocardial infarction. *Psychosom. Med.*, **44**, 519–527.

59. El-Gatit, A.M. and Haw, M. (2003) Relationship between depression and non-adherence to anticoagulant therapy after valve replacement. *East Mediterr. Health J.*, **9**, 12–19.

60. Irvine, J., Baker, B., Smith, J. et al. (1999) Poor adherence to placebo or amiodarone therapy predicts mortality: results from the CAMIAT

study. Canadian Amiodarone Myocardial Infarction Arrhythmia Trial. *Psychosom. Med.*, **61**, 566–575.

61. Granger, B.B., Swedberg, K., Ekman, I. et al. (2005) Adherence to candesartan and placebo and outcomes in chronic heart failure in the CHARM programme: double-blind, randomised, controlled clinical trial. *Lancet*, **366**, 2005–2011.

62. Simpson, S.H., Eurich, D.T., Majumdar, S.R. et al. (2006) A meta-analysis of the association between adherence to drug therapy and mortality. *BMJ*, **333**, 15.

63. Chao, J., Nau, D.P., Aikens, J.E. and Taylor, S.D. (2005) The mediating role of health beliefs in the relationship between depressive symptoms and medication adherence in persons with diabetes. *Res. Social Adm. Pharm.*, **1**, 508–525.

64. Krishnan, K.R., George, L.K., Pieper, C.F. et al. (1998) Depression and social support in elderly patients with cardiac disease. *Am. Heart J.*, **136**, 491–495.

65. Berkman, L.F. (1995) The role of social relations in health promotion. *Psychosom. Med.*, **57**, 245–254.

66. King, K.B. (1997) Psychologic and social aspects of cardiovascular disease. *Ann. Behav. Med.*, **19**, 264–270.

67. Brummett, B.H., Barefoot, J.C., Siegler, I.C. et al. (2001) Character-istics of socially isolated patients with coronary artery disease who are at elevated risk for mortality. *Psychosom. Med.*, **63**, 267–272.

68. Burg, M.M., Barefoot, J., Berkman, L. et al. (2005) Low perceived social support and post–myocardial infarction prognosis in the Enhanc-ing Recovery in Coronary Heart Disease Clinical Trial: the effects of treatment. *Psychosom. Med.*, **67**, 879–888.

69. Ruberman, W., Weinblatt, E., Goldberg, J.D. and Chaudhary, B.S. (1984) Psychosocial influences on mortality after myocardial infarc-tion. *N. Engl. J. Med.*, **311**, 552–559.

70. Case, R.B., Moss, A.J., Case, N. et al. (1992) Living alone after myocardial infarction. *JAMA*, **267**, 515–519.

71. Schmaltz, H.N., Southern, D., Ghali, W.A. et al. (2007) Living alone, patient sex and mortality after acute myocardial infarction. *J. Gen. Intern. Med.*, **22**, 572–578.

72. Frasure-Smith, N., Lespérance, F., Juneau, M. et al. (1999) Gender, depression, and one-year prognosis after myocardial infarction. *Psychosom. Med.*, **61**, 26–37.

73. Gersh, B.J. and Anderson, J.L. (1993) Thrombolysis and myocardial salvage; results of clinical trials and the animal paradigm – paradoxic or predictable? *Circulation*, **88**, 296–306.

74. Newby, L.K., Rutsch, W.R., Califf, R.M. et al. (1996) Time from symptom onset to treatment and outcomes after thrombolytic therapy. *J. Am. Coll. Cardiol.*, **27**, 1646–1655.

75. Fibrinolytic Therapy Trialists' (FTT) Collaborative Group (1994) Indications for fibrinolytic therapy and suspected acute myocardial infarction: collaborative overview of early mortality and major morbidity results from all randomised trials of more than 1000 patients. *Lancet*, **343**, 311–322.

76. De Luca, G., Suryapranata, H., Ottervanger, J.P. and Antman, E.M. (2004) Time delay to treatment and mortality in primary angioplasty for acute myocardial infarction: every minute of delay counts. *Circulation*, **109**, 1223–1225.

77. Brodie, B.R., Webb, J., Cox, D.A. et al. (2007) Impact of time to treatment on myocardial reperfusion and infarct size with primary percutaneous coronary intervention for acute myocardial infarction (from the EMERALD Trial). *Am. J. Cardiol.*, **99**, 1680–1686.

78. Frasure-Smith, N., Lesperance, F., Gravel, G. et al. (2000) Social support, depression, and mortality during the first year after myocardial infarction. *Circulation*, **101**, 1919–1924.

79. Matthews, S.C., Nelesen, R.A. and Dimsdale, J.E. (2005) Depressive symptoms are associated with increased systemic vascular resistance to stress. *Psychosom. Med.*, **67**, 509–513.

80. Taylor, C.B., Conrad, A., Wilhelm, F.H., et al. (2006) Psychophysiological and cortisol responses to psychological stress in depressed and nondepressed older men and women with elevated cardiovascular disease risk. *Psychosom. Med.*, **68**, 538–546.

81. Salomon, K., Clift, A., Karlsdóttir, M. and Rottenberg, J. (2009) Major depressive disorder is associated with attenuated cardiovascular reactivity and impaired recovery among those free of cardiovascular disease. *Health Psychol.*, **28**, 157–165.

82. York, K.M., Hassan, M., Li, Q. et al. (2007) Coronary artery disease and depression: patients with more depressive symptoms have lower cardiovascular reactivity during laboratory-induced mental stress. *Psychosom. Med.*, **69**, 521–528.

83. Carney, R.M., Freedland, K.E. and Veith, R.C. (2005) Depression, the autonomic nervous system, and coronary heart disease. *Psychosom. Med.*, **67** (Suppl.), S29–S33.

84. Veith, R.C., Lewis, N., Linares, O.A. et al. (1994) Sympathetic nervous system activity in major depression: basal and desipramine-induced alterations in plasma norepinephrine kinetics. *Arch. Gen. Psychiatry*, **51**, 411–422.

85. Lake, C., Pickar, D., Ziegler, M. et al. (1982) High plasma norepinephrine levels in patients with major affective disorder. *Am. J. Psychiatry*, **139,** 1315–1318.

86. Young, E.A., Lopez, J.F., Murphy-Weinberg, V. et al. (2000) Hormonal evidence for altered responsiveness to social stress in major depression. *Neuropsychopharmacology*, **23,** 411–418.

87. Mausbach, B., Dimsdale, J., Ziegler, M. et al. (2005) Depressive symptoms predict norepinephrine response to a psychological stressor task in Alzheimer's caregivers. *Psychosom. Med.*, **67,** 638–642.

88. Carney, R.M., Freedland, K.E., Veith, R.C. et al. (1999) Major depression, heart rate and plasma norepinephrine in patients with coronary heart disease. *Biol. Psychiatry*, **45,** 458–463.

89. Charney, D.S., Heninger, G.R., Sternberg, D.E. et al. (1982) Adrenergic receptor sensitivity in depression. Effects of clonidine in depressed patients and healthy subjects. *Arch. Gen. Psychiatry*, **39,** 290–294.

90. Mills, P.J., Adler, K.A., Dimsdale, J.E. et al. (2004) Vulnerable caregivers of Alzheimer disease patients have a deficit in β2-adrenergic receptor sensitivity and density. *Am. J. Geriatr. Psychiatry*, **12,** 281–286.

91. Wood, K., Whiting, K. and Coppen, A. (1986) Lymphocyte beta-adrenergic receptor density of patients with recurrent affective illness. *J. Affect. Disord.*, **10,** 3–8.

92. Jeanningros, R., Mazzola, P., Azorin, J.M. et al. (1991) Beta-adrenoceptor density of intact mononuclear leukocytes in subgroups of depressive disorders. *Biol. Psychiatry*, **15,** 789–798.

93. De Paermentier, F., Cheetham, S.C., Crompton, M.R. et al. (1990) Brain beta-adrenoceptor binding sites in antidepressant-free suicide victims. *Brain Res.*, **525,** 71–77.

94. Barton, D.A., Dawood, T., Lambert, E.A. et al. (2007) Sympathetic activity in major depressive disorder: identifying those at increased cardiac risk? *J. Hypertens.*, **25,** 2117–2124.

95. DiIorio, C., Shafer, P.O., Letz, R. et al. (2006) Behavioral, social, and affective factors associated with self-efficacy for self-management among people with epilepsy. *Epilepsy Behav.*, **9,** 158–163.

96. Maly, M.R., Costigan, P.A. and Olney, S.J. (2006) Determinants of self efficacy for physical tasks in people with knee osteoarthritis. *Arthritis Rheum.*, **55,** 94–101.

97. Turner, J.A., Ersek, M. and Kemp, C. (2005) Self-efficacy for managing pain is associated with disability, depression, and pain coping among retirement community residents with chronic pain. *J. Pain*, **6,** 471–479.

98. Sullivan, M.D., LaCroix, A.Z., Russo, J. and Katon, W.J. (1998) Self-efficacy and self-reported functional status in coronary heart disease: a six-month prospective study. *Psychosom. Med.*, **60**, 473–478.

99. Sarkar, U., Ali, S. and Whooley, M.A. (2007) Self-efficacy and health status in patients with coronary heart disease: findings from the Heart and Soul Study. *Psychosom. Med.*, **69**, 306–312.

100. Sarkar, U., Ali, S. and Whooley, M.A. (2009) Self-efficacy as a marker of cardiac function and predictor of heart failure hospitalization and mortality in patients with stable coronary heart disease: findings from the Heart and Soul Study. *Health Psychol.*, **28**, 166–173.

101. Ni, H., Nauman, D., Burgess, D. et al. (1999) Factors influencing knowledge of and adherence to selfcare among patients with heart failure. *Arch. Intern. Med.*, **159**, 1613–1619.

102. Barnason, S., Zimmerman, L., Nieveen, J. et al. (2003) Impact of a home communication intervention for coronary artery bypass graft patients with ischemic heart failure on self-efficacy, coronary disease risk factor modification, and functioning. *Heart Lung*, **32**, 147–158.

103. Dallow, C.B. and Anderson, J. (2003) Using self-efficacy and a trans-theoretical model to develop a physical activity intervention for obese women. *Am. J. Health Promot.*, **17**, 373–381.

104. Warnecke, R.B., Morera, O., Turner, L. et al. (2001) Changes in self-efficacy and readiness for smoking cessation among women with high school or less education. *J. Health Soc. Behav.*, **42**, 97–110.

105. Forgas, J.P., Bower, G.H. and Moylan, S.J. (1990) Praise or blame? Affective influences on attributions for achievement. *J. Pers. Soc. Psychol.*, **59**, 809–819.

106. Salovey, P. and Birnbaum, D. (1989) Influence of mood on health-relevant cognitions. *J. Pers. Soc. Psychol.*, **57**, 539–551.

CHAPTER 5

Depression and Cardiovascular Disease: The Safety of Antidepressant Drugs and their Ability to Improve Mood and Reduce Medical Morbidity

Alexander H. Glassman

Department of Clinical Psychopharmacology, New York State Psychiatric Institute, New York, NY, USA and Department of Psychiatry, Columbia University College of Physicians and Surgeons, New York, NY, USA

J. Thomas Bigger, Jr.

Department of Medicine, Columbia University College of Physicians and Surgeons, New York, NY, USA

Studies examining the potential relationship between heart disease and depression initially used community samples followed for extended periods of time [1, 2]. This approach had the advantage over clinical samples of avoiding confounding the diagnosis of depression

Depression and Heart Disease Edited by Alexander Glassman, Mario Maj and Norman Sartorius
© 2011 John Wiley & Sons, Ltd

with the effects of drugs used to treat the disorder. Community samples also had the advantage of avoiding the concern that depression resulted from pre-existing cardiovascular disease (CVD). In early community samples, few patients had either treated depression or symptomatic cardiac disease.

In the late 1980s, a scientist at Washington University in St. Louis suggested that using patients with pre-existing CVD, rather than excluding them, would reduce the sample size as well as the duration of follow-up required to identify an association between depression and cardiac disease [3]. Frasure-Smith et al. [4] used this approach in their landmark paper in 1993. They recruited 222 consecutive post myocardial infarction (MI) patients in a cardiac intensive care unit, administered a structured psychiatric interview and followed them for 6 months. Patients with a comorbid diagnosis of depression had a 16% 6-month mortality rate compared with 4% mortality rate in patients free of depression. After adjusting for the severity of the infarct and cardiac risk factors, the hazard ratio was 4.29 (95% CI 3.14, 5.44; $p = 0.013$). Unlike physically healthy patients with major depressive disorder, those with post-infarction depression had a 400% increase in the risk of dying (Figure 5.1).

Although it would take a number of years to firmly establish this threefold increase risk of dying, as well as the difference between physically healthy depressed patients followed over time and depressed post-MI patients [5, 6], it immediately raised the question

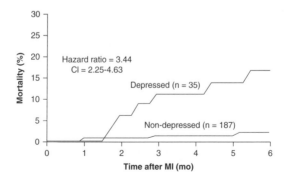

Figure 5.1 Cumulative mortality in depressed and non-depressed patients following myocardial infarction (MI) (adapted from Lesperance et al. [31]).

whether treatment of depression would reduce the markedly increased cardiac risk seen in post-MI patients.

Efforts to answer that question faced several major problems. Compared with testing the ability of an antidepressant to improve depressed mood, a very large sample size is required to test the effect of antidepressant therapy on mortality rates. If the mortality rate among depressed post-MI patients remained at 15%, a 20% reduction in mortality (the difference between 15% and 12% mortality) would require more than 4000 depressed post-MI patients to have adequate power to find a mortality difference if it were present. Although a 10% or 20% improvement in depression is a small effect, a 10% or 20% reduction in mortality would be clinically important. In addition, the Frasure-Smith observation occurred at just the time that medical therapy of coronary events was rapidly reducing mortality rates. It was unlikely that subsequent post-MI depression studies would find the same mortality rate that the Canadian investigators had originally observed [4].

Beyond the problem of sample size, there was a significant problem of safety. Although antidepressant drugs seemed like the most practical means of treating a large number of patients across a variety of medical settings, in the mid-1990s there were no data available on the safety of any antidepressant when given in the period immediately after an infarction.

THE SAFETY OF ANTIDEPRESSANT DRUGS

Prior to any definitive trial testing of whether antidepressant treatment would reduce mortality, it was necessary to establish the safety of antidepressant drugs in the immediate post-MI period. The safety data available at the time came from patients with stable heart disease, but suggested that selective serotonin reuptake inhibitors (SSRIs) were less likely to have cardiotoxicity than tricyclic antidepressants [7, 8].

The first adequately powered SSRI safety study in a post-MI population was the Sertraline Antidepressant Heart Attack Randomised Trial (SADHART) [9]. Following an initial feasibility study [10], SADHART began in 1997 and was published in 2002 [9]. A power analysis based on left ventricular ejection fraction (LVEF) indicated that a sample of 400 depressed post-MI patients would be required. A total of 369 were actually recruited and randomly assigned to treatment with placebo or sertraline. Absolutely no evidence of harm was found. After 16 weeks of treatment, LVEF measurements were almost identical in the sertraline and placebo groups. Similarly, heart rate, blood pressure (both systolic and diastolic), electrocardiogram (ECG) (PR, QRS and QTc), and 24-hour Holter ECG recordings were essentially identical.

An earlier small European study randomised 54 post-MI patients to either fluoxetine or placebo and also found that echocardiographic variables and the electrocardiographic variables heart rate, PR interval, QRS interval and QTc interval did not change during the acute treatment [11].

THE ABILITY OF ANTIDEPRESSANT DRUGS TO INFLUENCE MEDICAL MORBIDITY AND MORTALITY

The most surprising observation in SADHART [9] was a numerical reduction in the number of life-threatening cardiovascular events. The original hope was to test whether antidepressant treatment would reduce mortality. However, when the power analysis suggested that more than 4000 depressed post-MI patients would be required, that goal was entirely unrealistic. Cardiologists frequently used what is referred to as combined endpoints in order to reduce the sample size required and increase the chances that a trial can actually be completed. Even using a combined endpoint of death and recurrent MI, power analysis suggested that a sample of at least 2000 depressed post-MI patients would be required. Exposing that number of patients to a drug without specific evidence of safety could not be justified. Establishing safety was a prerequisite and a safety study with less than 20% of that sample was very unlikely to reveal any possible reduction in medical morbidity or mortality. Nevertheless, five life-threatening events were specified *a priori* and an events committee reviewed and adjudicated all severe adverse events. The prespecified events were mortality, stroke, recurrent MI, hospitalisation for angina and hospitalisation for heart failure. In every case, these prespecified life-threatening events occurred less frequently in the sertraline group.

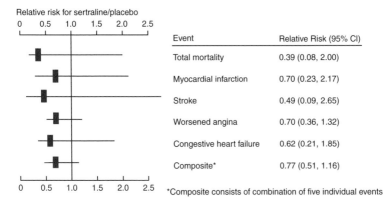

Figure 5.2 Relative risk (95% CI) for cardiovascular events: sertraline vs placebo (adapted from Glassman et al. [9]).

It is important to note that, although this decrease in combined risk was over 20%, it was not statistically significant (Figure 5.2).

Although intriguing, SADHARTs ability to test the reduction in life-threatening events was severely underpowered and was unable to prove that an SSRI could reduce adverse medical events. However, it did make it extremely unlikely that SSRIs caused adverse medical events.

About the same time that SADHART was testing the safety of sertraline in depressed post-MI patients, the National Heart, Lung, and Blood Institute (NHLBI) was testing the ability of psychotherapy to reduce cardiovascular outcomes in the same patient population. Because psychotherapy did not pose a safety risk, the investigators were able to institute treatment in all depressed post-MI patients without safety concerns inherent in drug treatment. Like SADHART, their power analysis suggested that about 2000 patients would be necessary if they used a combined endpoint of death and recurrent MI. The trial, Enhancing Recovery in Coronary Heart Disease (ENRICHD), tested psychotherapy against usual care [12]. They used a version of Beck's cognitive behavioural therapy (CBT) for depression as their active treatment [13]. ENRICHD was published the year after SADHART and, like sertraline, CBT had a modest beneficial effect on depression, but it had absolutely no effect on mortality.

However, it became an unexpected source of support for the possible beneficial effect of an SSRI on adverse medical events.

Although designed as a study of psychotherapy, ethics boards required that patients with a baseline Hamilton depression score equal to or greater than 24 be offered an antidepressant drug. They also required that patients who failed to respond after 5 weeks be offered antidepressant drug therapy and that, if a patient's physician thought that an antidepressant was required, that treatment should be given. As a result, although primarily a trial of psychotherapy, 301 of the 1834 depressed patients were treated with an SSRI. There was a significant reduction in the relative risk of death or recurrent MI (0.57; 95% CI 0.38, 0.84) in patients treated with SSRI after adjusting for disease severity and other factors. Although the observation came from a large sample and was highly statistically significant, patients were not randomly assigned to an antidepressant drug or placebo. In addition, 145 patients received an antidepressant other than an SSRI and, although not statistically significant, they also had a reduced risk of death or recurrent MI [14] (Table 5.1).

Taken together, SADHART and ENRICHD suggest, but do not prove, that antidepressant drug therapy in general, and SSRI treatment in particular, improve cardiovascular outcomes in depressed post-acute coronary syndrome (ACS) patients. The reduction in the rate of death or recurrent MI was similar and large in both ENRICHD and SADHART. However, SADHART was underpowered to detect a reduction in cardiovascular outcomes, and the number of actual deaths and recurrent MIs was small. In addition, because it was designed as a safety study, patients were administered blinded drug or placebo for only 6 months. Six months' exposure was adequate for evaluation of drug safety, but was a relatively short period of time to test if the drug reduces mortality.

Seven years after the initial trial, SADHART participants were re-examined for long-term mortality. After the 6 months of placebo controlled treatment, the treatment status of the participants was not known. The apparent reduction in mortality during the first 6 months of placebo-controlled treatment did not persist over the subsequent years [15]. However, patients who remained depressed at the end of 6 months, whether on drug or placebo, died twice as often as those who responded over the next 7 years.

Table 5.1 Effects of antidepressant drug use on clinical events over 30 months during the ENRICHD trial (adapted from Taylor et al. [14])

Variable	No antidepressant use (N = 1388)	Any antidepressant use (N = 446)	Type of antidepressant use	
			SSRI (N = 301)	Other (N = 145)
Death or recurrent MI				
Patients, no. (%)	361 (26.0)	96 (21.5)	59 (19.6)	37 (25.5)
HR (95% CI)				
Unadjusted	1.00	0.66 (0.43, 0.91)	0.61 (0.41, 0.90)	0.79 (0.48, 1.28)
Adjusted*	1.00	0.61 (0.45, 0.84)	0.57 (0.38, 0.84)	0.72 (0.44, 1.18)
All-cause mortality				
Patients, no. (%)	222 (16.0)	35 (7.8)	21 (7.0)	14 (9.7)
HR (95% CI)				
Unadjusted	1.00	0.72 (0.48, 1.06)	0.69 (0.43, 1.10)	0.72 (0.38, 1.35)
Adjusted*	1.00	0.63 (0.43, 0.93)	0.59 (0.37, 0.96)	0.64 (034, 1.22)
Recurrent MI				
Patients, no. (%)	205 (14.8)	73 (16.4)	45 (15.0)	28 (19.3)
HR (36% CI)				
Unadjusted	1.00	0.63 (0.41, 0.95)	0.58 (0.34, 0.97)	0.80 (0.42, 1.50)
Adjusted*	1.00	0.57 (0.38, 0.87)	0.53 (0.32, 0.90)	073 (0.38, 1.38)

CI – confidence interval; HR – hazard ratio; MI – myocardial infarction; SSRI – selective serotonin reuptake inhibitor.
*Multivariable model incorporating baseline age, baseline Beck Depression Inventory score, Killip class, ejection fraction, creatinine value, previous MI and prior diagnosis of congestive heart failure, stroke or transient ischaemic attack, pulmonary disease or diabetes mellitus.

ENRICHD followed patients for 30 months and, although *post hoc* and not randomised by drug treatment, did have information on whether or not participants were receiving antidepressants. The apparent benefit was striking (adjusted HR 0.57; 95% CI 0.38, 0.84) [14]. In addition to supporting the idea that SSRIs reduce death and recurrent MI, ENRICHD supplies further evidence of the safety of SSRIs in post-MI patients [12]. The ultimate marker for safety is mortality, and the fact that antidepressant-treated patients have a significantly reduced risk of death and recurrent MI is strong evidence that these drugs are not dangerous in post-MI patients.

There is a third post-MI trial, which the authors describe as an effectiveness study rather than an efficacy study, that compared the effects of an active treatment strategy with usual care. That study, the Myocardial INfarction and Depression – Intervention Trial (MIND–IT), used a randomised controlled design to test whether antidepressant treatment for post-MI depression improved long-term depression status and cardiovascular prognosis [16]. The study design was complex and the results were expressed in terms of the intervention group (N = 209) compared with usual care (N = 122). However, in the intervention group, 47 originally received mirtazapine and 44 received placebo. Patients from either group who had not responded after 8 weeks were treated with citalopram. In addition, 40 of the intervention group received non-pharmacological treatments and 45 received no treatment at all. Thus, the intervention groups included at least mirtazapine, citalopram, some non-pharmacological treatment plus 45 patients who received no treatment. SADHART and ENRICHD data suggested that any beneficial effect on medical outcome was present only during active treatment. In MIND-IT, both depression and cardiovascular outcomes were measured at 18 months, but there is no indication of how much time during those months the patients in any group were receiving any specific treatment. If any specific drug had an effect on either depression or cardiovascular outcomes, it could easily be obscured if all treatments did not have the same outcome.

When clinical trial data are not available, epidemiological studies, although never definitive, can sometimes be reassuring. However, even large epidemiological studies of depression and antidepressant treatment are not usually informative, because they confound the effects of depression and antidepressant treatment. Whether examining community samples, clinical, or specific post-MI or ACS populations, the association of antidepressant drugs with medical outcome is problematic. Patients who are treated with antidepressant drugs are much more likely to have depression than those who are not treated, and depression in untreated community samples has been shown to increase cardiovascular morbidity and mortality [1]. However, there is one Finnish cohort study in which all subjects without psychosis, hospitalised because of a suicide attempt from 1 January 1997 to 31 December 2003, were followed up through a nationwide computerised database [17]. The purpose of this study was not to examine the relationship between depression and cardiac mortality, but rather to look at the relationship between antidepressant use and suicide. Suicides are rare events, but prior suicide attempts are a major risk factor for future suicide attempts. By selecting patients who had a prior suicide attempt, the investigators greatly increased the chance that they could see an effect of antidepressants on suicide if one existed and antidepressants reduced the number of subsequent successful suicides. However, unexpectedly, 'antidepressant use, and especially SSRI use, was associated with a marked reduction in total mortality (-49%, $p < 0.001$), mostly attributable to a decrease in cardiovascular deaths'. The study involved 15 390 patients with a mean follow-up of 3.4 years and 'mortality during the use of tricyclic antidepressants (amitriptyline or doxepin), SSRIs (fluoxetine, citalopram, paroxetine, sertraline, or fluvoxamine), and SNAs (mianserin, mirtazapine, or venlafaxine) or other antidepressants was compared with the hazard during no antidepressant use'. Thus, the study had the advantage of a very large patient sample, but avoided the confounding of depression and antidepressant treatment, because all patients suffered from depression. This epidemiological survey involved over 50 000 patient/years and the observations are consistent with the magnitude of the reduction seen both in ENRICHD and SADHART.

IMPLEMENTING TREATMENT OF DEPRESSION IN A MEDICAL SETTING

A summary of the available evidence strongly suggests that SSRIs are safe in the immediate post-MI period and that both SSRIs and psychotherapy are effective antidepressants in post-MI patients. Although evidence suggests that the antidepressant benefit comes primarily from the more severely depressed segment of the post-MI major depressive disorder sample [18], it is premature to conclude that there is no treatment effect in the less severely depressed post-MI patients. Clinical trial comparisons in post-MI major depression, particularly a safety trial like SADHART, involve a control group that of necessity receives far more attention than ever occurs in usual care. That level of attention would almost certainly be interpreted by the patient as supportive and may have substantial therapeutic value.

The issue of whether treating post-MI depression reduces cardiovascular morbidity and mortality is complex. There is a strong suggestion that antidepressant drugs in general, and SSRIs in particular, reduce morbidity and mortality [19]. However, if SSRI treatment reduces morbidity and mortality, there is no evidence that any survival benefit occurs because these drugs are antidepressant. It could be that SSRIs reduce morbidity and mortality in all post-MI patients whether or not they are depressed. In contrast, there is no evidence that moderate improvement in mood associated with psychotherapy produces even a modest reduction in death or recurrent MI [12]. However, this is difficult to reconcile with the observation that patients with major depression after ACS who remit or markedly improve during placebo treatment have better outcomes than those who do not, which suggests that improvement in major depression has survival benefit [15].

The reality is, in fact, even more convoluted. It has been traditional to ask what mechanism drives this association between depression and heart disease, or more specifically, in the post-MI situation, between depression and morbidity and mortality. One thing that can be said is that there is almost certainly no single driving force. Autonomic tone, platelet reactivity, inflammatory response, early experience and genetics have all been implicated in both depression and cardiovascular disease, and each may play a variable role in any given patient [20]. In any of these situations, an antidepressant drug might reduce the medical risk by altering the risk variable directly or by improving depression and secondarily improving the variable.

In addition to the potential for antidepressant drugs to reduce risk either primarily or secondarily via biological mechanisms,

antidepressant treatment, when successful, can alter health behaviours. A large number of studies have shown that in cardiovascular
patients depression interferes with compliance to the doctor's advice [21, 22]. Depressed patients are less likely to stop smoking [23],
to participate in rehabilitation [24] and to adhere to medication
regimes [21, 25]. There is overwhelming evidence that beta-blockers,
statins and antiplatelet drugs reduce morbidity and mortality following MI [26]. However, medications do not improve the patient's
prognosis unless the patient takes the medication. Recent data suggest
that compliance to prescribed medication improves after improvement in mood [15]. Improvement in compliance would tend to reduce
mortality and should occur with either psychotherapy or pharmacotherapy, but only in that portion of the patient population whose
depression gets better [27]. Improvement in more physiological risk
indicators, such as heart rate variability, might occur in antidepressant-
treated patients regardless of whether the patient got better or not [28].

Although the evidence that SSRIs reduce mortality is circumstan-
tial and does not rise to the level that it can be considered a standard of
care, our approach to the MI patient has entirely reversed itself from
where it was less than a decade ago. Throughout the 1990s and into the
early 2000s, post-MI patients who appeared depressed were not
treated with antidepressant drugs unless the depression was extremely
severe. The rationale was that most post-MI depressions are related to
the psychological and physiological stress of the coronary event and
will improve spontaneously. Thus, the danger of antidepressant drugs
in patients with cardiac disease can be avoided. Much of the evidence
for drug cardiotoxicity stemmed from studies on the older tricyclic
antidepressants [29]. Although the SSRIs seem to have different
characteristics in cardiovascular patients, there were absolutely no
data on what happened in the acute MI period until SADHART tested
safety in ACS patients.

Over the last 10 years, the degree to which depression is not just a
painful, disabling mood state, but a condition with serious implications for health behaviours has also become apparent. Even mild
depressions increase the risk of adverse medical outcomes [30, 31].
Our group has recently published data from a 7-year follow-up of
SADHART participants looking at early predictors of long-term
mortality. The baseline severity of depression was associated with

an almost twofold increase in long-term mortality [32]. However, less intuitively, the failure of depression to remit by 6 months also predicted a doubling of mortality independent of the baseline severity. Although it is not clear that more aggressive antidepressant treatment of these non-responsive individuals would reduce mortality, it is obvious that they are at higher cardiovascular risk and should be treated with an aggressive medical regime by their physician.

Given that SSRI treatment of depression in the post-ACS period is safe, effective in reducing depressed mood, able to improve health behaviours and may reduce subsequent cardiac morbidity and mortality, it would seem obvious that treating depression is strongly indicated. However, the vast majority of post-ACS patients will not see a psychiatrically trained professional and many cases are not identified [33]. Patients as well as physicians frequently feel that it is reasonable to be depressed following a coronary event. In addition, cardiologists are often preoccupied with the immediate medical issues, and exploring the patient's mood state is not uppermost in their mind at that moment. The American Heart Association (AHA) recently published a scientific advisory [34] recommending the use of depression screening instruments and discussed utilisation of the two-question Patient Health Questionnaire (PHQ-2) [35]. This asks about the frequency of depressed mood and anhedonia over the prior 2 weeks, scoring each from 0 ('not at all') to 3 ('nearly every day'). A PHQ-2 score of ≥ 3 had a sensitivity of 83% and a specificity of 92% for major depression. If a PHQ-2 score is ≥ 3, the AHA recommended that a full PHQ-9 be obtained. Most patients can complete this without assistance in ≤ 5 min, and this assessment provides the sensitivity and specificity suitable for assigning a provisional diagnosis of major depression and a symptom severity score that can be used to identify patients for further evaluation and to make decisions about therapy.

Although the use of the PHQ or other screening instruments will improve the recognition of depression, studies have made it clear that recognition alone has very modest, if any, impact on depression outcome. Screening procedures need to be tied to some organised structure designed specifically to make sure that treatment is undertaken, pursued and modified when necessary. This approach is frequently referred to as 'collaborative care'. A recent example is the Prevention of Suicide in Primary Care Elderly: Collaborative Trial (PROSPECT) [36]. This trial evaluated the impact of a care management intervention on suicidal ideation and depression in older primary care patients and reported outcomes that occurred during a 2-year follow-up. PROSPECT screened 9072 patients of 20 primary care practices to find 599 study participants who were ≥60 years of age with major or minor depression. Participants were randomly assigned to either the PROSPECT collaborative intervention or usual care. The intervention consisted of services rendered by trained care managers, who offered algorithm-based recommendations to physicians and helped patients with treatment adherence during the 24-month trial. Compared with usual care, patients receiving the intervention were more likely to receive antidepressants and/or psychotherapy and had a 2.2 times greater decline in suicidal ideation over 24 months. Amongst patients with major depression, a significantly greater percentage of the intervention group achieved complete remission than in the usual-care group at 4, 8 and 24 months. However, patients with minor depression had favourable outcomes regardless of treatment assignment.

Bypassing the Blues, the first study of collaborative care in cardiac patients, also demonstrated an advantage of collaborative care over usual care in depressed post-coronary bypass patients [37]. Although smaller ($N = 302$) than the PROSPECT, this study, in which care was delivered over the phone by nurse care managers, also found a substantial and statistically significant advantage for collaborative care.

The evidence that SSRIs are safe in patients with coronary artery disease and particularly in patients following coronary event comes from both clinical trials [9, 12] and epidemiological studies [17, 38]. SADHART was by far the largest placebo-controlled safety trial and measured heart rate, blood pressure, ECG, ejection fraction, Holter monitors and heart rate variability repeated over 16 weeks of treatment. It found no evidence of harm with sertraline [9]. There were a number of smaller clinical trials in patients with CVD [8, 16] and some included surrogate measures of cardiac function [11]. Although it is more informative about safety to obtain surrogate measures such as blood pressure, ejection fraction or ventricular premature depolarisation, ultimately the gold standard for safety is adverse cardiac events.

For that reason, ENRICHD is very informative about SSRI safety even though no surrogate safety measures were obtained [12]. A total of 301 patients were treated with an SSRI (primarily sertraline) and those patients had a very significantly reduced rate of mortality and recurrent MI compared with the patients who were not drug treated. The only long-term cardiovascular risk associated with SSRIs has been the rare reports of upper gastrointestinal bleeding in older patients with known upper gastrointestinal disease [39]. Given the known antiplatelet effects of SSRIs, it is almost surprising that bleeding has been so uncommon a problem [40].

Amongst the SSRIs, the majority of the data have been obtained with sertraline and citalopram. It would seem very likely that escitalopram would have similar cardiac effects, although actual data are not available. The story is probably similar with fluoxetine and paroxetine; however, these two SSRIs have considerably more propensity to interact with other drugs than sertraline, citalopram or escitalopram. Ordinarily drug–drug interactions with SSRIs are not commonly problematic events. However, when treating the cardiac population, patients are often prescribed an extraordinary number of other drugs and the chances of meaningful drug–drug interactions escalate dramatically. In the SADHART study, the average post-MI patient was on 10 other medications.

It was not entirely surprising that SSRIs have proven to be safe in patients with cardiac disease. One of the marked differences between the SSRIs and the earlier tricyclic antidepressants is that the SSRIs do not cause cardiac death in overdose as the tricyclics do [41]. There has been literature that suggested that tricyclics even at therapeutic doses could be cardiotoxic and more problematic than SSRIs [42, 43]. What has been surprising is that both in the clinical trial data from ENRICHD and the epidemiological data from Finland, tricyclic treatment has also been associated with a decreased risk of mortality.

The US Preventive Services Task Force report [33] recommends that, when a patient screens positive for depression, a primary care provider familiar with managing depression and a case manager with a mental health background should follow and support that patient, and regular supervision of the case manager by a psychiatrist or psychologist should be available.

CONCLUSIONS

That depression is associated with cardiovascular morbidity and mortality is no longer open to question. Similarly, there is no question that the risk of morbidity and mortality increases with increasing severity of depression. Questions remain about the mechanisms that underlie this association, whether all types of depression carry the same degree of risk and to what degree treating depression reduces that risk.

There is no question that the benefits of treating depression associated with coronary artery disease far outweigh the risks. However, it remains true that depression following a coronary event is often not recognised. Even when recognised, it is often dismissed as understandable. There is a need to educate physicians and establish a system to identify, treat and follow up cardiac patients with depression. This is a major public health issue. In the United States there are over a half-million hospitalisations for myocardial infarction and probably more than that for unstable angina [44, 45] annually. Approximately 20% of these 1 million hospitalised cardiac patients will suffer from major depression, while an equal number will meet criteria for minor depression [46]. Thus, there are approximately 200 000 ACS patients each year who are at increased risk because of depression.

Given the low risk of SSRI treatment, the painful nature of depression and the multiple ways in which depression interferes with medical treatment regimens, it seems appropriate if there is any uncertainty about treatment to go ahead and treat. However, only a large definitive clinical trial, exploring if SSRI treatment of post-ACS depression reduces mortality, will motivate general medicine to identify and aggressively treat depression, and that type of trial is badly needed.

ACKNOWLEDGEMENT

The authors acknowledge support by the National Alliance for Research in Schizophrenia and Depression (NARSAD), the Suzanne C. Murphy Foundation and the Thomas and Caroline Royster Research Fund.

REFERENCES

1. Anda, R., Williamson, D., Jones, D. et al. (1993) Depressed affect, hopelessness, and the risk of ischemic heart disease in a cohort of United States adults. *Epidemiology*, **4**, 285–293.
2. Murphy, J. (1990) Depression in the community: findings from the Stirling County Study. *Can. J. Psychiatry*, **35**, 390–396.
3. Carney, R.M., Rich, M.W., Freedland, K.E. et al. (1988) Major depressive disorder predicts cardiac events in patients with coronary artery disease. *Psychosom. Med.*, **50**, 627–633.
4. Frasure-Smith, N., Lesperance, F. and Talajic, M. (1993) Depression following myocardial infarction. Impact on 6-month survival. *JAMA*, **270**, 1819–1825.
5. Bush, D.E., Ziegelstein, R.C., Patel, U.V. et al. (2005) *Post-Myocardial Infarction Depression*, Agency for Health Research and Quality, Rockville.
6. Wulsin, L.R. and Singal, B.M. (2003) Do depressive symptoms increase the risk for the onset of coronary disease? A systematic quantitative review. *Psychosom. Med.*, **65**, 201–210.
7. Roose, S.P., Glassman, A.H., Attia, E. and Woodring, S. (1994) Comparative efficacy of selective serotonin reuptake inhibitors and tricyclics in the treatment of melancholia. *Am. J. Psychiatry*, **151**, 1735–1739.
8. Roose, S.P., Glassman, A.H., Attia, E. et al. (1998) Cardiovascular effects of fluoxetine in depressed patients with heart disease. *Am. J. Psychiatry*, **155**, 660–665.
9. Glassman, A.H., O'Connor, C.M., Califf, R.M. et al. (2002) Sertraline treatment of major depression in patients with acute MI or unstable angina. *JAMA*, **288**, 701–709.
10. Shapiro, P.A., Lesperance, F., Frasure-Smith, N. et al. (1999) An open-label preliminary trial of sertraline for treatment of major depression after acute myocardial infarction (the SADHAT Trial). Sertraline Anti-Depressant Heart Attack Trial. *Am. Heart J.*, **137**, 1100–1106.
11. Strik, J.J., Honig, A., Lousberg, R. et al. (2000) Efficacy and safety of fluoxetine in the treatment of patients with major depression after first myocardial infarction: findings from a double-blind, placebo-controlled trial. *Psychosom. Med.*, **62**, 783–789.
12. Berkman, L.F., Blumenthal, J., Burg, M. et al. (2003) Effects of treating depression and low perceived social support on clinical events after myocardial infarction: the Enhancing Recovery in Coronary Heart Disease Patients (ENRICHD) Randomized Trial. *JAMA*, **289**, 3106–3116.

13. Beck, A.T., Rush, A.J., Shaw, B.F. and Emory, G. (1979) *Cognitive Therapy for Depression*, Guilford, New York.

14. Taylor, C.B., Youngblood, M.E., Catellier, D. et al. (2005) Effects of antidepressant medication on morbidity and mortality in depressed patients after myocardial infarction. *Arch. Gen. Psychiatry*, **62,** 792–798.

15. Glassman, A.H., Bigger, J.T. Jr and Gaffney, M. (2009) Psychiatric characteristics associated with long-term mortality among 361 patients having an acute coronary syndrome and major depression: seven-year follow-up of SADHART participants. *Arch. Gen. Psychiatry*, **66,** 1022–1029.

16. Honig, A., Kuyper, A.M., Schene, A.H. et al. (2007) Treatment of post-myocardial infarction depressive disorder: a randomized, placebo-controlled trial with mirtazapine. *Psychosom. Med.*, **69,** 606–613.

17. Tiihonen, J., Lonnqvist, J., Wahlbeck, K. et al. (2006) Antidepressants and the risk of suicide, attempted suicide, and overall mortality in a nationwide cohort. *Arch. Gen. Psychiatry*, **63,** 1358–1367.

18. Glassman, A.H., Bigger, J.T. and Gaffney, M. (2006) Onset of major depression associated with acute coronary syndromes: relationship of onset, major depressive disorder history, and episode severity to sertraline benefit. *Arch. Gen. Psychiatry*, **63,** 283–288.

19. Glassman, A.H. and Bigger, J.T. Jr (2007) Antidepressants in coronary heart disease: SSRIs reduce depression, but do they save lives? *JAMA*, **297,** 411–412.

20. Skala, J.A., Freedland, K.E. and Carney, R.M. (2006) Coronary heart disease and depression: a review of recent mechanistic research. *Can. J. Psychiatry*, **51,** 738–745.

21. Carney, R.M., Freedland, K.E., Eisen, S.A. et al. (1995) Major depression and medication adherence in elderly patients with coronary artery disease. *Health Psychol.*, **14,** 88–90.

22. Ziegelstein, R.C., Fauerbach, J.A., Stevens, S.S. et al. (2000) Patients with depression are less likely to follow recommendations to reduce cardiac risk during recovery from a myocardial infarction. *Arch. Intern. Med.*, **160,** 1818–1823.

23. Holtrop, J.S., Stommel, M., Corser, W. and Holmes-Rovner, M. (2009) Predictors of smoking cessation and relapse after hospitalization for acute coronary syndrome. *J. Hosp. Med.*, **4,** E3–E9.

24. Casey, E., Hughes, J.W., Waechter, D. et al. (2008) Depression predicts failure to complete phase-II cardiac rehabilitation. *J. Behav. Med.*, **31,** 421–431.

25. DiMatteo, M.R., Lepper, H.S. and Croghan, T.W. (2000) Depression is a risk factor for noncompliance with medical treatment: meta-analysis of

the effects of anxiety and depression on patient adherence. *Arch. Intern. Med.*, **160**, 2101–2107.

26. Mukherjee, D., Fang, J., Chetcuti, S. et al. (2004) Impact of combination evidence-based medical therapy on mortality in patients with acute coronary syndromes. *Circulation*, **109**, 745–749.

27. Rieckmann, N., Gerin, W., Kronish, I.M. et al. (2006) Course of depressive symptoms and medication adherence after acute coronary syndromes – An electronic medication monitoring study. *J. Am. Coll. Cardiol.*, **48**, 2218–2222.

28. Glassman, A.H., Bigger, J.T., Gaffney, M. and Van Zyl, L.T. (2007) Heart rate variability in acute coronary syndrome patients with major depression: influence of sertraline and mood improvement. *Arch. Gen. Psychiatry*, **64**, 1025–1031.

29. Glassman, A.H., Roose, S.P. and Bigger, J.T. Jr (1993) The safety of tricyclic antidepressants in cardiac patients. Risk-benefit reconsidered. *JAMA*, **269**, 2673–2675.

30. Carney, R.M., Freedland, K.E., Steinmeyer, B. et al. (2008) Depression and five year survival following acute myocardial infarction: a prospective study. *J. Affect. Disord.*, **109**, 133–138.

31. Lesperance, F., Fräsure-Smith, N., Talajic, M. and Bourassa, M.G. (2002) Five-year risk of cardiac mortality in relation to initial severity and one-year changes in depression symptoms after myocardial infarction. *Circulation*, **105**, 1049–1053.

32. Glassman, A.H., Bigger, J.T. and Gaffney, M. (2009) Psychiatric characteristics associated with long-term mortality among 361 patients having an acute coronary syndrome and major depression. Seven-year follow-up of SADHART participants. *Arch. Gen. Psychiatry*, **66**, 1022–1029.

33. US. Preventive Services Task Force (2002) Screening for depression: recommendations and rationale. *Ann. Intern. Med.*, **136**, 760–764.

34. Lichtman, J.H., Bigger, J.T., Blumenthal, J.A. et al. (2008) Depression and coronary heart disease: recommendations for screening, referral, and treatment: a science advisory from the American Heart Association Prevention Committee of the Council on Cardiovascular Nursing, Council on Clinical Cardiology, Council on Epidemiology and Prevention, and Interdisciplinary Council on Quality of Care and Outcomes Research endorsed by the American Psychiatric Association. *Circulation*, **118**, 1768–1775.

35. Kroenke, K., Spitzer, R.L. and Williams, J.B. (2003) The Patient Health Questionnaire-2: validity of a two-item depression screener. *Med. Care*, **41**, 1284–1292.

36. Alexopoulos, G.S., Reynolds, C.F. 3rd, Bruce, M.L. et al. (2009) Reducing suicidal ideation and depression in older primary care patients: 24-month outcomes of the PROSPECT study. *Am. J. Psychiatry*, **166**, 882–890.

37. Rollman, B.L., Belnap, B.H., Lemenager, M.S. et al. (2009) Telephone-delivered collaborative care for treating post-CABG depression: a randomized controlled trial. *JAMA*, **302**, 2095–2103.

38. Haukka, J., Arffman, M., Partonen, T. et al. (2009) Antidepressant use and mortality in Finland: a register-linkage study from a nationwide cohort. *Eur. J. Clin. Pharmacol.*, **65**, 715–720.

39. Gasse, C., Christensen, S., Riis, A. et al. (2009) Preadmission use of SSRIs alone or in combination with NSAIDs and 30-day mortality after peptic ulcer bleeding. *Scand. J. Gastroenterol.*, **44**, 1288–1295.

40. Kim, D.H., Daskalakis, C., Whellan, D.J. et al. (2009) Safety of selective serotonin reuptake inhibitor in adults undergoing coronary artery bypass grafting. *Am. J. Cardiol.*, **103**, 1391–1395.

41. Glassman, A.H. and Davis, J.M. (1987) Overdose with tricyclic drugs. *Psychiatr. Ann.*, **17**, 410–411.

42. Glassman, A.H., Roose, S.P. and Bigger, J.T. Jr (1993) The safety of tricyclic antidepressants in cardiac patients – risk/benefit reconsidered. *JAMA*, **269**, 2673–2675.

43. Roose, S.P., Laghrissi-Thode, F., Kennedy, J.S. et al. (1998) Comparison of paroxetine and nortriptyline in depressed patients with ischemic heart disease. *JAMA*, **279**, 287–291.

44. Roger, V.L., Jacobsen, S.J., Weston, S.A. et al. (2002) Trends in the incidence and survival of patients with hospitalized myocardial infarction, Olmsted County, Minnesota, 1979 to 1994. *Ann. Intern. Med.*, **136**, 341–348.

45. Rosamond, W., Flegal, K., Furie, K. et al. (2008) Heart disease and stroke statistics – 2008 update: a report from the American Heart Association Statistics Committee and Stroke Statistics Subcommittee. *Circulation*, **117**, e25–e146.

46. Thombs, B.D., Bass, E.B., Ford, D.E. et al. (2006) Prevalence of depression in survivors of acute myocardial infarction. *J. Gen. Intern. Med.*, **21**, 30–38.

CHAPTER 6

Psychotherapies for Depression in People with Heart Disease

Robert M. Carney and Kenneth E. Freedland

*Department of Psychiatry, Washington University School of Medicine,
St. Louis, MO, USA*

Research on psychotherapy for depression began decades ago, but the first major clinical trials of psychotherapy for depression in patients with heart disease did not appear until the 1990s. Recent trials have tested several psychotherapeutic interventions for comorbid depression in heart disease. Although there have been very few head-to-head comparisons, some of these interventions have fared better than others in randomised controlled trials (RCTs). On the other hand, none of them has proven to be as highly or as uniformly efficacious as one might hope. Consequently, clinical researchers are searching for ways to increase the efficacy of these interventions and to deliver them more effectively and efficiently.

There has been much less interest in developing completely new forms of therapy for depressed cardiac patients, since fundamental paradigm shifts have been very rare in the history of psychotherapy research. Despite the limitations of the current generation of psychotherapies, interest in translation and dissemination of clinical trial findings has been growing along with an increasing awareness among cardiologists, primary care physicians and other health care providers

Depression and Heart Disease   Edited by Alexander Glassman, Mario Maj and Norman Sartorius
© 2011 John Wiley & Sons, Ltd

that depression is both prevalent and consequential in patients with heart disease.

This chapter summarises the current state of clinical research on some of the most promising forms of psychotherapy for depression in patients with heart disease. In general, the interventions that have been tested to date were 'borrowed' in the sense that they were originally developed for depressed but otherwise medically well patients and are now being applied to patients who are both depressed and medically ill. The interventions for cardiac patients are not very different from those originally designed for healthier patients, but some have been modified or extended in various ways to address the unique needs and problems of depressed patients with heart disease.

Although several different psychotherapeutic interventions for depression have been tested in cardiac patient populations, they are not entirely distinct from one another. The commonalities among them are not limited to the non-specific factors that are shared by virtually all forms of psychotherapy, such as clinical attention in the context of a supportive, therapeutic relationship. They extend to specific therapeutic objectives and techniques. For example, techniques designed to build problem-solving skills are obviously central to problem-solving therapy (PST), but they also play an important role in cognitive behaviour therapy (CBT).

Several other overriding issues should also be taken into account in reviewing this literature. First, major systems of psychotherapy such as CBT encompass multiple techniques and strategies. Consequently, the cognitive behavioural intervention that is tested in one RCT may differ in important ways from the one that is tested in another. Second, depression is a complex disorder in patients with heart disease, and the stressors that contribute to it are complex as well. In contrast to the highly structured treatment manuals that have been developed for more circumscribed interventions such as smoking cessation, depression treatment manuals tend to permit considerable individualisation of treatment, as well as clinical flexibility on the part of the therapist, in order to accommodate the complexity of the target condition. This means that, even within the experimental arm of a single trial, the intervention is likely to differ from one patient to the next. Third, there are considerable differences in training, experience, competence and interpersonal skills among therapists. These differences can affect treatment planning and implementation, and they can moderate the outcomes of psychotherapy. Fourth, efficacy is determined not only by the potency of the experimental intervention employed in a RCT, but of the control condition as well [1]. Control conditions in this area of research can be as complex as the experimental interventions themselves. Finally, it is impossible to conduct double-blind trials of psychotherapeutic interventions: the participants are informed at enrolment as to the groups to which they may be randomly assigned and, after randomisation, they know which one they were assigned to. Even the most rigorous psychotherapy trials are only single-blind.

COGNITIVE BEHAVIOUR THERAPY

Historical Background

During the 1960s and 1970s, clinical scientists began to apply findings from laboratory research on animal behaviour to problematic human behaviours. An approach known as behaviour modification [2, 3] grew out of B.F. Skinner's laboratory research on operant behaviour [4], that is observable actions that are controlled by their environmental consequences. A broader approach that came to be known as behaviour therapy incorporated principles derived from research on classical (Pavlovian) conditioning and on social learning, in addition to operant behaviour [5, 6].

Early clinical behaviourists tended to eschew covert psychological phenomena such as thoughts, beliefs and feelings, and focused instead on observable and measurable behaviours. This served to distance the behaviour therapy movement from psychoanalysis and other forms of psychotherapy that were regarded as unscientific due to their emphasis on unobservable phenomena and untested (and perhaps even untestable) theories. Over time, however, behaviourally orientated clinicians and researchers found it increasingly difficult to ignore cognitions and emotions, particularly in treating conditions such as depression that have salient cognitive and emotional features. This led in 1970s to a 'cognitive revolution' in behaviour therapy. The publication of two of A.T. Beck's classic papers [7, 8] and his groundbreaking textbook *Cognitive Therapy of Depression* [9] were seminal events in cognitive revolution in depression treatment. Over the next three decades, a variety of other therapeutic models for depression and for many other conditions also blended cognitive, emotional and behavioural elements, and came to be known collectively as cognitive behavioural therapies [10]. The term 'cognitive therapy' *per se* is generally reserved for Beck's variety of CBT.

Cognitive therapy targets biased information processing, which, according to Beck's cognitive model, plays a central role in depression and other forms of emotional distress. Depressogenic biases are found in a variety of cognitive errors and dysfunctional thoughts, beliefs and attitudes [11]. During depressive episodes, for example, negative thoughts about oneself, one's personal world and the future are quite common, and they tend to produce dysphoria and feelings of hope-lessness. Cognitive therapy also uses cognitive and behavioural techniques to target other facets of depression, such as behavioural activation and activity scheduling to address inactivity and loss of interest or pleasure in usual activities; social skills training to address certain types of interpersonal difficulties; and coping and problem-solving skills training to improve the patient's ability to manage depressogenic stressors [9].

There has been much more research on cognitive-behavioural interventions than on any other form of psychotherapy, which helps to explain why many biobehavioural researchers have favoured CBT when choosing psychotherapeutic interventions to test in medically ill patient populations. A recent review of meta-analyses of CBT reported large effect sizes for some disorders and more moderate effects for others [12]. One of the most rigorous meta-analyses of CBT for unipolar depression in adults reported a large effect size (0.82) for comparisons with wait list or placebo controls, moderate effects for comparisons with antidepressants (0.38) and other miscellaneous psychotherapies (0.24), but little evidence of superiority (0.05) to other forms of behaviour therapy. Also, when the miscellaneous psychotherapies were restricted to comprehensive treatments for depression, the effect size dropped to 0.16 [13]. Thus, there is strong empirical support for the use of CBT for depression, but less support for its superiority to other well-tested psychotherapeutic interventions for depression.

Cognitive Therapy for Cardiac Patients

Enhancing Recovery in Coronary Heart Disease

The Enhancing Recovery in Coronary Heart Disease (ENRICHD) study was the first large RCT to test CBT for depression in a cardiac patient population. The participants were enrolled within 1 month of hospitalisation for an acute myocardial infarction (MI). The trial targeted two related psychosocial risk factors for post-MI morbidity and mortality, that is depression and low perceived social support (LPSS). To qualify on the basis of depression, patients had to meet the DSM-IV criteria for a current major depressive episode, or for minor depression with a past history of major depression, according to a structured interview [14]. The LPSS eligibility criteria were based on the ENRICHD Social Support Inventory (ESSI) [15].

The primary purpose of ENRICHD was to determine whether treatment of depression and/or LPSS decreases the risks of reinfarction and mortality after an acute MI. The primary composite endpoint was reinfarction or death from any cause. Depression and LPSS were intermediate targets and were considered to be secondary outcomes. In other words, ENRICHD was designed to test a mediation hypothesis, not to evaluate the efficacy of CBT for depression or LPSS *per se*.

In designing this sort of trial, it is advisable to choose an intervention that is already known to have a large effect on the intermediate target; otherwise, there is little chance of improving the primary medical outcome. Unfortunately, there had not been any RCTs of CBT for depression or LPSS in cardiac patients prior to ENRICHD, and the ENRICHD investigators had neither enough time nor sufficient resources to conduct preliminary tests of their intervention. Instead, they had to extrapolate from the existing literature on cognitive-behavioural interventions for depression and for social and interpersonal problems [16]. Patients with heart disease or other serious medical illnesses had been excluded from most of these trials. Consequently, there has been almost as much interest in the effects of the ENRICHD intervention on the trial's secondary (psychosocial) outcomes as in its primary medical endpoint.

Participants assigned to the intervention arm received up to 6 months of individual CBT. The therapists used J.S. Beck's *Cognitive*

Therapy: Basics and Beyond [17], A.T. Beck's *Cognitive Therapy of Depression* [9] and a study-specific treatment protocol [16] as their core treatment manuals. The Beck Institute for Cognitive Therapy and Research provided training and supervision. When feasible, the patients participated in cognitive-behavioural group therapy, in addition to individual CBT. Also, patients who were severely depressed, or who did not respond to the cognitive-behavioural intervention, were also offered sertraline.

The individual CBT sessions were supposed to be held on a weekly basis, although many patients had to skip some of their sessions due to illness, logistical problems such as a lack of transportation or competing demands. The treatment continued until 6 months had elapsed or until the patient met criteria for successful completion. These criteria, for depressed patients, required at least six therapy sessions, a score of ≤7 on the Beck Depression Inventory (BDI) and a score of 12 on the CBT Performance Criteria Scale (CBT-PCS) [18]. The therapists rated the patient's progress with respect to the following objectives: (a) utilisation of behavioural activation techniques; (b) ability to identify problematic situations and emotions; (c) ability to identify dysfunctional thoughts in problematic and/or emotionally arousing situations; (d) utilisation of cognitive-behavioural techniques to evaluate and modify dysfunctional thoughts and beliefs; (e) utilisation of cognitive-behavioural techniques for active problem-solving; and (f) ability to apply cognitive-behavioural skills to new and future problems and relapses [19]. These criteria reflect the fact that relapses are common in depression. Consequently, the aim of CBT is not only to hasten the end of the current depressive episode, but also to prevent relapses of depression in the short term and recurrences in the long term.

Of the 2481 patients who were enrolled in ENRICHD, 1238 were randomly assigned to the intervention arm and 1243 to the usual care (UC) control group. Approximately 40% of the participants in both arms were enrolled on the basis of depression alone, and about 35% had both depression and LPSS. The intervention began, on average, only 17 days after the MI (range 10–27 days). The median number of sessions was 11 (interquartile range 6–19), although patients with both depression and LPSS required more sessions (median 13; interquartile range 6–20) than those with only one psychosocial risk factor. Fewer than one-third of the intervention participants and only 25% of the depression-only patients received group therapy. In both of the depressed subgroups, 77% completed at least six sessions of CBT. In the depressed-only subgroup, 56% met the successful completion target for depression improvement and 47% met the CBT-PCS criteria. In the subgroup with both depression and LPSS, 43% met the improvement criteria and 41% met the CBT-PCS criteria. In short, while many patients responded very well to the intervention, some were still depressed and deficient in relevant cognitive-behavioural skills despite up to 6 months of treatment [20].

On the other hand, many of the patients who did not meet the criteria for successful completion had far fewer CBT sessions than were available to them. Some of them may not have been motivated to complete such an intensive and prolonged treatment programme. Others may have wanted more therapy than they received, but encountered barriers such as rehospitalisations, a scarcity of free time after returning to work or a lack of transportation. Consequently, the ENRICHD trial fostered interest in ways to increase motivation and to overcome barriers to psychotherapy for depressed medically ill patients.

The ENRICHD intervention was superior to usual care for depression, but only modestly. On the BDI, depressed participants in the intervention arm improved from an average of 17.7 ± 8.1 at baseline to 9.1 ± 8.6 at 6 months; in the UC arm, they went from 18.0 ± 8.6 to 12.2 ± 9.1. The between-group difference at 6 months was 2.7 points (95% CI 1.7, 3.7) in favour of the intervention. On the BDI, the severity of each symptom is rated on a 0–3 scale, with 0 representing absent and 3 representing severe. Thus, one way to judge the magnitude of the difference would be to think of the typical UC patient as having one more severe symptom of depression than the typical CBT patient, or for the former to have two or three mild symptoms that had been eliminated altogether in the latter.

The between-group difference in perceived social support was also fairly small at 6 months in ENRICHD. In light of the relatively modest effects on the targeted psychosocial risk factors, it is not surprising that there was no between-group difference in reinfarction-free survival [20]. However, a secondary analysis showed that patients with major depression who completed the 6-month intervention phase and whose depression improved had a lower risk of late mortality (i.e. starting 6 months after the index MI) than those who remained depressed despite completing the intervention. This suggests that treatment-resistant depression may pose a greater risk of mortality after an MI than does treatment-responsive depression. The effect might be due instead to other differences between patients who either do or do not respond to treatment. However, the hazard ratio remained significant after adjustment for demographic and medical predictors of all-cause mortality in ENRICHD [21, 22]. Another secondary analysis found no such benefit for improvement in perceived social support, despite the fact that LPSS at baseline predicted an increase risk of mortality [23].

As noted previously, participants in the intervention arm who were severely depressed or whose depression did not respond to CBT were offered sertraline. For a variety of reasons, including patient preference, some of the participants who were eligible for an antidepressant did not receive one [24]. Patients in the UC arm were free to consult their own physician about a prescription, if they so chose. At baseline, 4.8% of the UC group and 9.1% of the intervention group were already taking an antidepressant. By 6 months, antidepressant utilisation rose to 13.4% and 20.5% in the UC and CBT arms, respectively, and it further increased to 20.6% and 28% by the end of the 29-month (average) follow-up [20]. Thus, some of the depressed participants received CBT alone, and others received CBT augmented with an antidepressant medication. This was not determined by random assignment, and there were baseline differences between the patients who received an antidepressant and those who did not. This makes it very difficult to evaluate whether combination therapy was superior to CBT alone in ENRICHD.

A secondary analysis was conducted to identify predictors of psychosocial outcomes in the intervention arm. One of the aims of this analysis was to identify the 'active ingredients' of this multifaceted intervention. Another was to determine whether treatment outcomes were affected by individualisation of the intervention, and by variability in patient adherence (e.g. completion of CBT homework). Better depression outcomes were achieved by patients who received most or all of the depression-specific components of the cognitive-behavioural intervention, who also received the social communication and assertiveness components and who completed a high proportion of cognitive-behavioural homework assignments. A higher number of sessions and use of an antidepressant predicted worse depression outcomes, but these negative effects were confounded with the baseline severity of depression and did not reflect any adverse effects of treatment. Better social support outcomes were predicted by racial or ethnic minority status and by completing most of the homework assignments. None of the LPSS-specific components of the intervention predicted better perceived social support at 6 months. On the contrary, the social communication and assertiveness components were independent predictors of *worse* social support outcomes among patients with LPSS. Thus, although the standard ingredients of CBT for depression generalised very well to the treatment of depression in post-MI patients, the putative active ingredients of the intervention for LPSS apparently did not work as intended [25].

Finally, a recent secondary analysis was conducted to explore the effects of the ENRICHD cognitive-behavioural group intervention. Compared with the individual CBT-only participants, the group participants had somewhat better depression outcomes (BDI change from baseline to 6 months, -8.1 ± 9.2 vs -9.3 ± 9.2), but slightly worse social support outcomes (ESSI change from baseline to 6 months, 5.6 ± 6.5 vs 5.2 ± 6.2). No survival benefit of group CBT was evident after adjustment for confounders. Nevertheless, these results point to the need for more rigorous, prospective comparisons of group versus individual CBT for depression in cardiac patients [26].

Treatment of Depression After Coronary Artery Bypass Surgery

A recent RCT was the first study to test the efficacy of CBT for depression after coronary artery bypass graft (CABG) surgery [27]. One hundred and twenty-three patients (50% women, 19% racial minorities, mean age 61 years) were enrolled in the study and randomly assigned to 12 weeks of individual CBT, a supportive stress management (SSM) intervention or UC for depression. Although ENRICHD offered up to 6 months of CBT, this trial limited the intervention phase to 12 weeks. This was done primarily to facilitate participation in the post-treatment assessment session, by synchronising it with the patients' 3-month post-operative follow-up visit with their cardiac surgeon. Some patients might have achieved further gains if the treatment phase had been extended to 6 months. As discussed above, however, the median number of CBT sessions in ENRICHD was 11 for patients with depression alone and 13 for those with both depression and LPSS. Furthermore, many trials of CBT for unipolar depression have been limited to 12–16 weeks, and some have been as brief as 8 weeks. In this context, limiting the intervention to 12 weeks was clearly justifiable.

As in ENRICHD, A.T. Beck's *Cognitive Therapy of Depression* and J.S. Beck's *Cognitive Therapy: Basics and Beyond* were core CBT treatment manuals. In addition, the therapists also utilised two supplemental manuals: J.S. Beck's *Cognitive Therapy for Challenging Problems* [28] and *Heart Disease: Advances in Psychotherapy* by Skala et al. [29]. The cognitive-behavioural intervention was very similar to the one employed in ENRICHD, except that the shorter duration of treatment made it necessary to focus more intensively on the problems that seemed to be the most significant contributors to the patient's depression, and that were potentially modifiable within 12 weeks. A novel CBT Problem List form was developed for this trial to facilitate prioritisation of treatment objectives.

The SSM intervention was delivered in the setting of a supportive therapeutic relationship with the aim of improving the patient's skills for coping with stressful life events and daily stressors. The rationale for the intervention was that, if patients were better able to cope with the psychosocial stressors that contributed to initiate and/or maintain their depression, this should help to accelerate remission of depression. In addition, it is a less complex intervention than CBT, and it is compatible with the less intensive stress management programmes that are often provided to patients in the course of cardiac rehabilitation. The intervention applied well-established, manualised stress management techniques [30–32] to depressogenic stressors.

Approximately two-thirds of the participants met the DSM-IV criteria for a current major depressive at enrolment, and one-third met the criteria for minor depression. About 50% of the participants in all three arms of the study were taking non-study antidepressants at enrolment, and continued to do so throughout the trial.

The primary outcome of the trial was remission of depression, defined as a score of 7 or less on the 17-item Hamilton Rating Scale for Depression (HAM-D). The proportion of patients in remission at 3 months was significantly higher in the CBT (71%) and the SSM (57%) arms than in the UC arm (33%). The differences among the groups narrowed between 3 and 6 months, but the remission rates differed once again at 9 months (73%, 57% and 35% for the CBT, SSM and UC groups, respectively). In a covariate-adjusted analysis, continuous HAM-D scores were significantly lower at 3 months in the CBT (mean $\pm$ standard error 5.5 ± 1.0) and the SSM (7.8 ± 1.0) arms than in the UC arm (10.7 ± 1.0). CBT was superior to UC at most of the assessment visits on secondary measures of depression, anxiety, hopelessness, stress and health-related quality of life. In contrast, SSM was superior to UC only on some measures at some time points.

There were also differences between the CBT and SSM arms in the intensity and duration of treatment. Ninety-eight per cent of the CBT participants completed the intervention compared with only 79% of the SSM participants. CBT participants also attended an average of 11 sessions, compared with only eight for the SSM participants. The groups did not differ on the Burns Empathy Scale, a measure of the patient's perception of the quality of the therapeutic relationship, or on the Treatment Process Scale, a measure of the therapist's perception of the relationship. This pattern of findings suggests that, although the participants in both groups believed that the intervention was beneficial, the SSM participants tended to experience a sense of diminishing returns by the eighth session, if not sooner. This is not too surprising, in that SSM had a relatively narrow focus on coping with depressogenic stressors. CBT, in contrast, addressed a broader variety of target problems, and did so with a larger set of techniques and strategies.

One of the key limitations of this trial is that it was not adequately powered for direct comparisons of the CBT and SSM arms; it only had sufficient power to compare both active interventions with the UC control condition. Nevertheless, it is apparent that CBT had larger and more persistent effects on more of the outcomes of interest than did SSM. The main advantages of SSM are that it is less complex than CBT and that it apparently requires less time to complete.

Approximately half of the patients in all three arms were taking non-study antidepressants during the trial. When antidepressant use was included in the multivariable models, it did not predict better depression scores and it had no effect on most of the other secondary outcomes. The effects of CBT and SSM held up after adjustment for antidepressant use. Also, there was no evidence of an interaction between antidepressant use and treatment arm, which suggests that combination therapy was not superior to CBT or SSM alone. It is important to consider, however, that antidepressant use was not determined by random assignment, and that patients who were on an antidepressant had been taking it at a therapeutic dosage for at least 6 weeks at study enrolment. It is likely that some of these patients had benefited from the antidepressant, at least to some degree, despite the fact that they were still sufficiently depressed to qualify for the trial.

In summary, CBT appears to be a useful therapeutic option for patients who are depressed after CABG surgery, whether or not they are taking an antidepressant. In many cases, good outcomes can be achieved in 12 weeks. SSM also has some potential as an intervention for post-CABG depression, although it is probably not as efficacious as CBT.

INTERPERSONAL PSYCHOTHERAPY

Background

Interpersonal psychotherapy (IPT), developed in the 1980s by G. Klerman and M. Weissman, is a manualised, well-tested psychotherapeutic intervention for depression [33, 34]. It is a brief, highly structured intervention that focuses on interpersonal problems. In particular, it targets interpersonal conflicts, social role transitions, grief and interpersonal deficits. Although other problems, deficits and stressors often contribute to the onset and/or maintenance of depression, they are not addressed in IPT.

Unlike CBT, IPT is not based on a specific model of psychopathology, although it fits within a tradition of interpersonal and social approaches to psychotherapy that originated in H. S. Sullivan's classic work in the 1930s. Like CBT, IPT was originally developed as a treatment for depression, but has since been applied to other problems as well. Most of the therapeutic techniques used in IPT, such as supportive listening, clarification of the patient's interpersonal beliefs and encouragement of emotional expression, are not specific to that therapy; they are also used in other forms as psychotherapy. Because of its relatively narrow focus and its reliance on standard counselling techniques, IPT is thought to require less training, experience and clinical sophistication than does CBT.

IPT was superior to clinical management plus a pill placebo in the landmark Treatment of Depression Collaborative Research Program (TDCRP) [35, 36] and, among severely depressed patients, imipramine plus clinical management (CM) and IPT produced similar outcomes. IPT has demonstrated efficacy in other treatment and maintenance trials, including studies of recurrent major depression (e.g. [37, 38]), although other trials have failed to demonstrate the superiority of IPT over a control condition [39].

The CREATE Trial

The multicentre Canadian Cardiac Randomized Evaluation of Antidepressant and Psychotherapy Efficacy (CREATE) study [40, 41] was the first randomised trial of IPT for depression in patients with stable coronary artery disease (CAD). In addition to testing the efficacy of IPT, CREATE was also an antidepressant efficacy trial. These two objectives were accomplished in a single, 2×2 factorial, parallel-group, 12-week trial with a sample of 284 patients with CAD and comorbid major depression. A HAM-D score of 20 or higher was an eligibility requirement. Because patients with minor depression or with mild major depression were excluded, CREATE studied more severely depressed patients, on average, than ENRICHD. Another difference was that patients were recruited immediately after an acute MI for ENRICHD, but neither a recent nor a remote history of MI was required for CREATE. Approximately two-thirds of the CREATE sample had a previous MI at study enrolment.

All of the participants were randomised twice. First, they were randomly assigned to receive 12 weekly sessions of IPT plus CM, or CM alone. Second, they were randomised to 12 weeks of 20–40 mg of citalopram per day, or to a matching placebo. Thus, all participants received CM, and the factorial groups received IPT + citalopram +

CM, or IPT + pill placebo + CM, or citalopram + CM, or pill placebo + CM. The primary outcome measure was the change from baseline to 12 weeks on the 24-item version of the HAM-D, and the BDI-II was used as a secondary outcome measure.

IPT + CM was not superior to CM alone in CREATE. In fact, there was a trend in favour of CM on the HAM-D (mean HAM-D change, -2.26 points; 96.7% CI -4.78, 0.27). However, this trend was not apparent on the BDI-II (mean change, 1.13 points; 98.3% CI -1.90, 4.16). In contrast, citalopram was superior to pill placebo on both measures.

It is not entirely clear why IPT, which has demonstrated efficacy in at least some studies of depressed but medically well patients, had no apparent benefit in CREATE. However, it is important to take into account that CM was provided to all participants, including those who received IPT. Thus, this was not a test of IPT alone. In the IPT arm, the same therapist administered 20–25 min of CM, followed by IPT in the same sessions. The CM component was based primarily on the manualised CM approach utilised in the TDCRP trial [42]. It provided clinical attention, a review of symptoms, information about depression and its treatment, reassurance and encouragement to adhere to the study protocol.

A planned subgroup analysis showed that CM alone might be superior to IPT + CM for patients with inadequate social support and/ or significant functional impairment in daily activities. This suggests that IPT, which focuses on interpersonal problems, may not be well suited for depressed cardiac patients who also have poor social support or functional impairment.

This finding is reminiscent of the results of a secondary analysis of the TDCRP, which showed that *low* social dysfunction predicted superior response to IPT and that *low* cognitive dysfunction predicted superior response to CBT [43]. This was a surprising and counterintuitive finding for those who expected IPT to be especially well suited to patients with a high level of social dysfunction, and CBT to be especially efficacious for patients who have dysfunctional thoughts, beliefs or attitudes. It raised the possibility that these forms of psychotherapy may work best when they capitalise on patients' relative strengths, rather than focusing exclusively on their most salient psychosocial problems and deficits.

Also, as discussed previously, participants with low perceived social support who completed the ENRICHD intervention had somewhat better social support outcomes than those who were assigned to usual care, but the social support-specific ingredients of the intervention did not predict better social support outcomes.

Taken together, the CREATE and ENRICHD findings suggest that further psychotherapeutic treatment development research is needed to address social isolation, inadequate social support, interpersonal problems and other forms of social maladjustment, in both depressed and non-depressed cardiac patients. They also suggest that CBT may be a better choice than IPT for treating depression in patients with coronary disease. However, additional trials, including head-to-head comparisons, are still needed.

PROBLEM-SOLVING THERAPY

Background

PST was originally developed by D'Zurilla and co-workers [44, 45]. Nezu et al. [46] conducted some of the earliest PST trials and subsequently refined the intervention and extended it to a variety of patient populations.

PST is based on a model in which successful coping depends on two different attributes, that is problem orientation and problem-solving style. Problem orientation refers to beliefs and attitudes about problems in living and about one's ability to cope with them. The individual's problem orientation can be adaptive or maladaptive. For example, while some people are confident in their ability to solve problems and understand that successful problem-solving often takes initiative and effort, others lack confidence and believe that solutions depend more on luck, fate or other people's actions than on personal effort. Problem-solving style refers to the cognitive and behavioural activities in which one engages when confronted with problems in living. A rational problem-solving style is usually adaptive; in contrast, an avoidant, impulsive or careless style is often maladaptive. The goal of PST is to improve both the patient's problem orientation and his/her problem-solving style in order to improve his/her ability to cope with current and future problems. This, in turn, can help to decrease depression and other forms of emotional distress.

PST has been applied to a variety of problems, but is probably best known as a brief, efficient, structured intervention for depression that, like IPT, requires less extensive training and clinical experience than CBT to administer. Problem-solving and improving cognitive and behavioural problem-solving skills are also standard ingredients of CBT. Consequently, PST can be viewed as one of the components of more comprehensive CBT for depression. Recent meta-analytic reviews of PST have concluded that it is more efficacious than various control conditions, although it has not been shown to be superior to CBT or to other active interventions. However, these meta-analyses have also shown that there is considerable heterogeneity in outcomes among PST studies. A number of different factors may contribute to this heterogeneity, including the severity of depression. It appears that PST may be insufficient as a standalone intervention for severe depression, but that it can benefit patients with mild to moderate depression [47, 48].

The COPES Project

PST per se has not yet been subjected to a straightforward, randomised comparison with a control condition or with another active treatment for depression in cardiac patients. However, it performed well in the Improving Mood-Promoting Access to Collaborative Treatment (IMPACT) trial. IMPACT targeted depression in older adults with chronic medical conditions [49]. PST was subsequently employed in the Coronary Psychosocial Evaluation Studies (COPES) project [50]. The COPES study utilised a patient preference-driven, stepped care design in which PST was one of the first-line options within the intervention arm. Patients who preferred antidepressants but who had an inadequate response were also able to add or switch to PST. The results of COPES have not yet been published, but preliminary reports suggest that depressed patients with coronary disease who prefer PST tend to respond well to this form of psychotherapy.

DIRECTIONS FOR FUTURE RESEARCH

Two competing trends are emerging in research on psychotherapy for depression in cardiac patients. First, the few rigorous RCTs that have been conducted so far have shown that even the most efficacious of the current generation of interventions produce relatively modest outcomes. Thus, there are needs for treatment development research, for studies to differentiate between treatment-responsive and treatment-resistant forms of depression, and for efforts to adapt and extend existing depression interventions to meet the distinctive needs of specific cardiac patient populations. The overriding goal of this line of research is to increase the efficacy of psychotherapy for depression in cardiac patients. This is important not only to address depression *per se*, but it is also a critical prerequisite for future efforts to determine whether treatment of depression can improve medical outcomes and reduce the risk of mortality in cardiac patients.

Second, there is a growing recognition that, even if an intervention is highly efficacious, it may be difficult to translate into clinical practice if it requires intensive or extensive contacts with a highly trained, experienced, clinically sophisticated psychotherapist. It can even be difficult to implement such interventions in the setting of carefully controlled, randomised efficacy trials. Consequently, there are efforts to develop simpler, more efficient interventions that can be delivered by a wider variety of interventionists.

Some of the early attempts to do this provided brief, in-hospital counselling and psychoeducational programs for patients recovering from an acute MI [51, 52], but interest in this strategy has decreased along with the typical length of stay for MI patients. One of the strategies that is gaining interest among clinical researchers is to employ specific components of a more comprehensive cognitive-behavioural approach for outpatients. PST is one example. Another is to extract the behavioural activation (BA) component of CBT and use it as a standalone treatment for depression. Standalone BA has not been systematically tested yet in cardiac patients, but it is appealing because productive, recreational, and social activities are meaningful targets of treatment in their own right in cardiac patients. BA has been evaluated in quite a few studies of depressed but medically well patients. A recent meta-analysis showed that it tends to have relatively strong effects in comparison to control conditions and that its efficacy is comparable to that of more comprehensive CBT for depression [53].

Another strategy is to deliver existing interventions in ways that are more convenient for patients. For example, some studies have utilised group therapies which enable therapists to treat multiple patients at the same time [26, 54]. Others have delivered psychotherapy or counselling interventions via telephone, either alone or in combination with other treatment components [26, 54–57]. Telephone-delivered CBT has compared favourably with in-person CBT in recent studies [58, 59]. Thus, it may be possible to identify interventions that are more efficient or convenient, that require less clinical skill to deliver, or that are less expensive than CBT for depression, without sacrificing efficacy in the process. Again, however, there is considerable room to improve the efficacy of even the most elaborate, expensive, and potent of the currently available interventions for depression in patients with heart disease.

Efforts to include psychotherapy within multifaceted approaches to depression care have also provided impetus to the search for efficient yet efficacious interventions. Stepped care for depression, as tested in the COPES trial, is one approach. Collaborative care is another. In a recent trial, nurses provided brief depression counselling in conjunction with self-help materials within a collaborative care intervention for depression after CABG surgery [60, 61]. Still another is to take patient preference into account and offer psychotherapy as one of two or more treatment options. This approach was utilised in the COPES trial, as well as in the European Myocardial Infarction and Depression Intervention Trial (MIND-IT) [62].

As noted previously, the appearance of a radically new form of psychotherapy is a rare development. Consequently, over the coming decade, efforts to increase the efficacy and/or efficiency of psychotherapeutic interventions will focus primarily on cognitive-behavioural, interpersonal, and other existing treatment paradigms. For example, a promising direction in mainstream psychotherapy research has involved a search for underlying factors that contribute to treatment efficacy, regardless of the specific 'brand' of psychotherapy [63]. As another example, we are currently conducting a trial in which CBT for depression is integrated with a cognitive-behavioural intervention for improving self-care of heart failure. Depression and poor self-care are mutually reinforcing problems in heart failure [64], so extending CBT in this manner has the potential to yield better depression outcomes as well as better functional outcomes in this patient population.

Although much more work remains to be done in this area, enough is already known about psychotherapy for comorbid depression in heart disease to suggest that a higher priority should be placed on translation of this research into clinical practice. In many cases, cardiac patients do not receive any treatment for their depression. Most of those who are treated receive an antidepressant, but relatively few receive CBT, IPT, or PST. Although many patients respond very well to antidepressants, some do not [65]. Many depressed cardiac patients could benefit from evidence-based psychotherapeutic interventions, either alone or in combination with antidepressants.

REFERENCES

1. Mohr, D.C., Spring, B., Freedland, K.E. et al. (2009) The selection and design of control conditions for randomized controlled trials of psychological interventions. *Psychother. Psychosom.*, **78**, 275–284.
2. Krasner, L., Bandura, A. and Ullmann, L.P. (1965) *Research in Behavior Modification: New Developments and Implications*, Holt, Rinehart and Winston, New York.
3. Ullmann, L.P. and Krasner, L. (1965) *Case Studies in Behavior Modification*, Holt, Rinehart and Winston, New York.
4. Skinner, B.F. (1953) *Science and Human Behavior*, Macmillan, New York.
5. Bandura, A. (1977) *Social Learning Theory*, Prentice Hall, Englewood Cliffs.
6. Wolpe, J. (1969) *The Practice of Behavior Therapy*, 1st edn, Pergamon, New York.
7. Beck, A.T. (1963) Thinking and depression. I. Idiosyncratic content and cognitive distortions. *Arch. Gen. Psychiatry*, **9**, 324–333.
8. Beck, A.T. (1964) Thinking and depression. II. Theory and therapy. *Arch. Gen. Psychiatry*, **10**, 561–571.
9. Beck, A.T., Rush, A.J., Shaw, B.F. and Emery, G. (1979) *Cognitive Therapy of Depression*, Guilford, New York.

10. Dobson, K.S. (2009) *Handbook of Cognitive Behavioral Therapies*, 3rd edn, Guilford, New York.

11. Beck, A.T. (2005) The current state of cognitive therapy: a 40-year retrospective. *Arch. Gen. Psychiatry*, **62,** 953–959.

12. Butler, A.C., Chapman, J.E., Forman, E.M. and Beck, A.T. (2006) The empirical status of cognitive-behavioral therapy: a review of meta-analyses. *Clin. Psychol. Rev.*, **26,** 17–31.

13. Wampold, B.E., Minami, T., Baskin, T.W. and Callen, T.S. (2002) A meta-(re)analysis of the effects of cognitive therapy versus 'other therapies' for depression. *J. Affect. Disord.*, **68,** 159–165.

14. Freedland, K.E., Skala, J.A., Carney, R.M. et al. (2002) The Depression Interview and Structured Hamilton (DISH): rationale, development, characteristics, and clinical validity. *Psychosom. Med.*, **64,** 897–905.

15. Mitchell, P.H., Powell, L., Blumenthal, J. et al. (2003) A short social support measure for patients recovering from myocardial infarction: the ENRICHD Social Support Inventory. *J. Cardiopulm. Rehabil.*, **23,** 398–403.

16. ENRICHD Investigators (2001) Enhancing Recovery in Coronary Heart Disease (ENRICHD) study intervention: rationale and design. *Psychosom. Med.*, **63,** 747–755.

17. Beck, J.S. (1995) *Cognitive Therapy: Basics and Beyond*, Guilford, New York.

18. Freedland, K.E. and Beck, J.S. (1995) *CBT Performance Criteria Scale*.

19. ENRICHD Investigators (1998). *ENRICHD manual of operations, Vol. 2*, ENRICHD Coordinating Center, Chapel Hill, NC.

20. Berkman, L.F., Blumenthal, J., Burg, M. et al. (2003) Effects of treating depression and low perceived social support on clinical events after myocardial infarction: the Enhancing Recovery in Coronary Heart Disease Patients (ENRICHD) Randomized Trial. *JAMA*, **289,** 3106–3116.

21. Carney, R.M., Blumenthal, J.A., Freedland, K.E. et al. (2004) Depression and late mortality after myocardial infarction in the Enhancing Recovery in Coronary Heart Disease (ENRICHD) study. *Psychosom. Med.*, **66,** 466–474.

22. Jaffe, A.S., Krumholz, H.M., Catellier, D.J. et al. (2006) Prediction of medical morbidity and mortality after acute myocardial infarction in patients at increased psychosocial risk in the Enhancing Recovery in Coronary Heart Disease Patients (ENRICHD) study. *Am. Heart J.*, **152,** 126–135.

23. Burg, M.M., Barefoot, J., Berkman, L. et al. (2005) Low perceived social support and post-myocardial infarction prognosis in the Enhancing

Recovery in Coronary Heart Disease clinical trial: the effects of treatment. *Psychosom. Med.*, **67,** 879–888.

24. Taylor, C.B., Youngblood, M.E., Catellier, D. et al. (2005) Effects of antidepressant medication on morbidity and mortality in depressed patients after myocardial infarction. *Arch. Gen. Psychiatry*, **62,** 792–798.

25. Cowan, M.J., Freedland, K.E., Burg, M.M. et al. (2008) Predictors of treatment response for depression and inadequate social support – the ENRICHD randomized clinical trial. *Psychother. Psychosom.*, **77,** 27–37.

26. Saab, P.G., Bang, H., Williams, R.B. et al. (2009) The impact of cognitive behavioral group training on event-free survival in patients with myocardial infarction: the ENRICHD experience. *J. Psychosom. Res.*, **67,** 45–56.

27. Freedland, K.E., Skala, J.A., Carney, R.M. et al. (2009) Treatment of depression after coronary artery bypass surgery: a randomized controlled trial. *Arch. Gen. Psychiatry*, **66,** 387–396.

28. Beck, J.S. (2005) *Cognitive Therapy for Challenging Problems: What to do when the Basics Don't Work*, Guilford, New York.

29. Skala, J.A., Freedland, K.E. and Carney, R.M. (2005) *Heart Disease: Advances in Psychotherapy – Evidence-Based Practice*, Hogrefe & Huber, Cambridge.

30. Bernstein, D.A. and Borkovec, T.D. (1973) *Progressive Relaxation Training: A Manual for the Helping Professions*, Research Press, Champaign.

31. Bernstein, D.A., Borkovec, T.D. and Hazlett-Stevens, H. (2000) *New Directions in Progressive Relaxation Training: A Guidebook for Helping Professionals*, Praeger, Westport, CN.

32. Smith, J.C. (2002) *Stress Management: A Comprehensive Handbook of Techniques and Strategies*, Springer, New York.

33. Klerman, G.L. (1984) *Interpersonal Psychotherapy of Depression*, Basic Books, New York.

34. Weissman, M.M., Markowitz, J.C. and Klerman, G.L. (2000) *Comprehensive Guide to Interpersonal Psychotherapy*, Basic Books, New York.

35. Elkin, I., Shea, M.T., Watkins, J.T. et al. (1989) National Institute of Mental Health Treatment of Depression Collaborative Research Program. General effectiveness of treatments. *Arch. Gen. Psychiatry*, **46,** 971–982.

36. Shea, M.T., Elkin, I., Imber, S.D. et al. (1992) Course of depressive symptoms over follow-up. Findings from the National Institute of

Mental Health Treatment of Depression Collaborative Research Program. *Arch. Gen. Psychiatry*, **49,** 782–787.

37. Frank, E., Kupfer, D.J., Perel, J.M. et al. (1990) Three-year outcomes for maintenance therapies in recurrent depression. *Arch. Gen. Psychiatry*, **47,** 1093–1099.

38. Kupfer, D.J., Frank, E., Perel, J.M. et al. (1992) Five-year outcome for maintenance therapies in recurrent depression. *Arch. Gen. Psychiatry*, **49,** 769–773.

39. de Mello, M.F., de Jesus, M.J., Bacaltchuk, J. et al. (2005) A systematic review of research findings on the efficacy of interpersonal therapy for depressive disorders. *Eur. Arch. Psychiatry Clin. Neurosci.*, **255,** 75–82.

40. Frasure-Smith, N., Koszycki, D., Swenson, J.R. et al. (2006) Design and rationale for a randomized, controlled trial of interpersonal psychotherapy and citalopram for depression in coronary artery disease (CREATE). *Psychosom. Med.*, **68,** 87–93.

41. Lesperance, F., Frasure-Smith, N., Koszycki, D. et al. (2007) Effects of citalopram and interpersonal psychotherapy on depression in patients with coronary artery disease: the Canadian Cardiac Randomized Evaluation of Antidepressant and Psychotherapy Efficacy (CREATE) trial. *JAMA*, **297,** 367–379.

42. Fawcett, J., Epstein, P., Fiester, S.J. et al. (1987) Clinical management–imipramine/placebo administration manual. NIMH Treatment of Depression Collaborative Research Program. *Psychopharmacol. Bull.*, **23,** 309–324.

43. Sotsky, S.M., Glass, D.R., Shea, M.T. et al. (1991) Patient predictors of response to psychotherapy and pharmacotherapy: findings in the NIMH Treatment of Depression Collaborative Research Program. *Am. J. Psychiatry*, **148,** 997–1008.

44. D'Zurilla, T.J. and Goldfried, M.R. (1971) Problem-solving and behavioral intervention. *J. Abnorm. Psychol.*, **78,** 107–126.

45. D'Zurilla, T.J. and Nezu, A.M. (2007) *Problem-Solving Therapy: A Positive Approach to Clinical Intervention*, 3rd edn, Springer, New York.

46. Nezu, A.M., Nezu, C.M. and Perri, M.G. (1989) *Problem-Solving Therapy for Depression: Theory, Research, and Clinical Guidelines*, John Wiley & Sons Inc., New York.

47. Cuijpers, P., van Straten, A. and Warmerdam, L. (2007) Problem solving therapies for depression: a meta-analysis. *Eur. Psychiatry*, **22,** 9–15.

48. Malouff, J.M., Thorsteinsson, E.B. and Schutte, N.S. (2007) The efficacy of problem solving therapy in reducing mental and physical health problems: a meta-analysis. *Clin. Psychol. Rev.*, **27,** 46–57.

49. Harpole, L.H., Williams, J.W. Jr, Olsen, M.K. et al. (2005) Improving depression outcomes in older adults with comorbid medical illness. *Gen. Hosp. Psychiatry*, **27**, 4–12.

50. Burg, M.M., Lesperance, F., Rieckmann, N. et al. (2008) Treating persistent depressive symptoms in post-ACS patients: the project COPES phase-I randomized controlled trial. *Contemp. Clin. Trials*, **29**, 231–240.

51. Thompson, D.R. and Meddis, R. (1990) A prospective evaluation of in-hospital counselling for first time myocardial infarction men. *J. Psychosom. Res.*, **34**, 237–248.

52. Oldenburg, B., Perkins, R.J. and Andrews, G. (1985) Controlled trial of psychological intervention in myocardial infarction. *J. Consult. Clin. Psychol.*, **53**, 852–859.

53. Mazzucchelli, T., Kane, R. and Rees, C. (2009) Behavioral activation treatments for depression in adults: a meta-analysis and review. *Clin. Psychol. Sci. Pract.*, **16**, 383–411.

54. Appels, A., van Elderen, T., Bar, F. et al. (2006) Effects of a behavioural intervention on quality of life and related variables in angioplasty patients: results of the EXhaustion Intervention Trial. *J. Psychosom. Res.*, **61**, 1–7.

55. McLaughlin, T.J., Aupont, O., Bambauer, K.Z. et al. (2005) Improving psychologic adjustment to chronic illness in cardiac patients. The role of depression and anxiety. *J. Gen. Intern. Med.*, **20**, 1084–1090.

56. Lewin, R.J., Coulton, S., Frizelle, D.J. et al. (2009) A brief cognitive behavioural preimplantation and rehabilitation programme for patients receiving an implantable cardioverter-defibrillator improves physical health and reduces psychological morbidity and unplanned readmissions. *Heart*, **95**, 63–69.

57. Simon, G.E., Ludman, E.J., Tutty, S. et al. (2004) Telephone psychotherapy and telephone care management for primary care patients starting antidepressant treatment: a randomized controlled trial. *JAMA*, **292**, 935–942.

58. Mohr, D.C., Vella, L., Hart, S. et al. (2010) The effect of telephone-administered psychotherapy on symptoms of depression and attrition: a meta-analysis. *Clin. Psychol. Sci. Pract.*, **15**, 243–253.

59. Mohr, D.C., Hart, S.L., Julian, L. et al. (2005) Telephone-administered psychotherapy for depression. *Arch. Gen. Psychiatry*, **62**, 1007–1014.

60. Rollman, B.L., Belnap, B.H., LeMenager, M.S. et al. (2009) The Bypassing the Blues treatment protocol: stepped collaborative care for treating post-CABG depression. *Psychosom. Med.*, **71**, 217–230.

61. Rollman, B.L., Belnap, B.H., LeMenager, M.S. et al. (2009) Telephone-delivered collaborative care for treating post-CABG depression: a randomized controlled trial. *JAMA*, **302**, 2095–2103.

62. van Melle, J.P., de Jonge, P., Honig, A. et al. (2007) Effects of antidepressant treatment following myocardial infarction. *Br. J. Psychiatry*, **190**, 460–466.

63. Beutler, L.E. (2009) Making science matter in clinical practice: redefining psychotherapy. *Clin. Psychol. Sci. Pract.*, **16**, 301–317.

64. Riegel, B., Moser, D.K., Anker, S.D. et al. (2009) State of the science: promoting self-care in persons with heart failure: a scientific statement from the American Heart Association. *Circulation*, **120**, 1141–1163.

65. Glassman, A.H., O'Connor, C.M., Califf, R.M. et al. (2002) Sertraline treatment of major depression in patients with acute MI or unstable angina. *JAMA*, **288**, 701–709.

Acknowledgement

The World Psychiatric Association gratefully acknowledges the support of the following donors for this initiative: the Lugli Foundation in Rome, the Italian Society of Biological Psychiatry, Eli Lilly and Bristol-Myers Squibb.

Index

Page numbers in *italics* refer to Figures; those in **bold** to Tables.

Depression and Heart Disease   Edited by Alexander Glassman, Mario Maj and Norman Sartorius
© 2011 John Wiley & Sons, Ltd

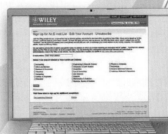